For Sandy and Niki

A Change in Fashion

Susan Gale

A Change in Fashion

Susan Gale

Copyright © 2013 Susan Gale

ISBN: 978-0-9576584-0-0

This book is published by Susan Gale Publishing in conjunction with WRITERSWORLD, and is produced entirely in the UK. It is available to order from most bookshops in the United Kingdom, and is also globally available via UK based Internet book retailers.

Copy edited by Sue Croft

Cover design by Jag Lall

Cover images from dreamstime.com

WRITERSWORLD
2 Bear Close Flats,
Bear Close, Woodstock
Oxfordshire,
OX20 1JX,
UnitedKingdom
☎ 01993 812500
☎ +44 1993 812500

www.writersworld.co.uk

The text pages of this book are produced via an independent certification process that ensures the trees from which the paper is produced come from well managed sources that exclude the risk of using illegally logged timber while leaving options to use post-consumer recycled paper as well.

ONE

Paris, Spring 1967

Rays of bright sunshine blinking through the carriage window revealed criss-crossing rail intersections, station platforms flashing past and an ever-tightening grid of cables overhead as the train clattered towards its final destination. The door of the compartment slid open.

"Les billets, s'il vous plaît." The ticket inspector pushed back his peaked cap and reached for the metal clippers that dangled on a chain from his belt. His glance fell on the slim hand with its long ringless fingers handing him two tickets, then rose to meet a pair of warm hazel eyes set wide apart in an oval face framed by smooth dark hair.

"Merci, mademoiselle." He punched the tickets and handed them back.

"Merci, monsieur." Her lips curved in a smile that made him pause for a moment. He had been working on the Calais-Paris route long enough to recognize British travellers, but in this case he was unsure. Her creamy complexion had the glow of an Englishwoman's and her soft voice could have betrayed a slight accent, but her appearance had a flair that was decidedly Parisian.

Holly waited until he had slid the door shut behind him.

"The sketches won't need much more than touching up, madame. I'll finish them tonight so that you can take them with you to the office in the morning. That way we should just manage to make the deadline for the May issue." Steadying her notebook against one knee as the train swung into a long bend, she frowned slightly. Deftly she added a few strokes of her pencil before handing the pages to the elegantly dressed woman sitting opposite.

Arlette de Châtigny smiled at the enthusiasm of her young travelling companion. The trip to London had been worthwhile but arduous, allowing them only two days for Mary Quant, Biba and other exciting designers in Kensington and Chelsea. Holly's sketches sparkled with their bright, innovative ideas. Arlette's practised eye fell on the uppermost one: a narrow black dress devoid of any detail and outrageously short, worn with thigh-high patent leather boots. Devastatingly simple, it would shock the established fashion industry of Paris to its conservative roots. This was what she had been waiting for.

As fashion editor of *Mode et Beauté*, France's most popular magazine for women, Arlette was always on the look-out for new impulses. She longed to take French fashion out of the hands of middle-aged men who designed with wealthy middle-aged women in mind, men for whom sales figures and balance sheets were more important than the women who wore their clothes, men who failed to realize that young working women needed creative but inexpensive fashion to match the lives they led. This breath of English air on the Parisian fashion scene would raise a storm.

Arlette passed the sketches back and Holly laid them carefully inside her portfolio. The train was slowing down. As the platform of the Gare du Nord slipped into view, she rose and struggled to remove Arlette's Vuitton travelling bag and her own worn suitcase from the luggage rack. Arlette pulled down the window with one gloved hand and, with the other holding her black pill-box hat tightly over her chignon, she leant out as far as possible.

"Henri! Henri! Nous voici!" Despite his years, an elderly grey-uniformed chauffeur sprinted along the platform beside them as the train ground to a halt. He swung the heavy carriage door open and helped Arlette to alight before turning to relieve Holly of their baggage.

'Les voyageurs à destination de Londres sont priés de . . . '

The voice that droned mechanically from the station loudspeaker was suddenly drowned by the metallic clatter of a trolley loaded with luggage that swept past. As Holly followed the other travellers thronging towards the exit gate, the sounds drew her thoughts back to the day when she had arrived in Paris for the first time. She could once again physically feel Arlette's letter in her hand. Suddenly overcome by the enormity of the step she had taken, she had not dared to let go of it for a moment in this city where she was completely alone.

'Madame de Châtigny thanks you for your application and, having checked your excellent references, is delighted to offer you the post as au pair for her daughter.'

The closing phrases conveying the writer's expression of respect, so strangely formal and quite unlike the French she had learned at school, had given her the first indication that she was about to enter a different world.

Sinking into the soft leather in the back of the silver Citröen Déesse, Holly was glad that Arlette had become engrossed in a lively conversation with Henri on the subject of the unusually mild spring weather. While the limousine purred along the boulevards, she relived her first impressions of this loveliest of cities. So different from the peace and solitude of her Yorkshire moorland home, its sights and sounds had overwhelmed her, numbing her brain. Was this the rush hour or was the traffic always so dense? Cars and taxis, vans and lorries jostled for the right of way, brakes screeching, horns blasting, drivers cursing as they jockeyed for position. Only the imperturbable calm of the chauffeur, who had maintained a dignified silence in the midst of the chaos, had allowed her to relax sufficiently to become aware of her surroundings. She could still remember her first glimpse of the stately white buildings, the balconies with their delicately-wrought balustrades, elegant in their uniformity, the wide pavements with their scurrying passers-by and crowded open-air cafés, and everywhere the fresh green tracery of spring foliage. Had it really been two years ago? It seemed like yesterday.

Suddenly there was a glitter of sun on water; the Seine lay before them. As on that first occasion, Holly caught her breath when the cathedral of Notre Dame rose like a magnificent ship from its island in the river. The car slowed to walking pace, weaving to avoid tangled groups of tourists as it crossed the narrow bridge leading to the Ile Saint-Louis, the quieter of the two islands, hiding behind its famous sister, the Ile de la Cité.

They had left the boulevards behind them now. Tall, classical façades fronted narrow streets, cutting out much of the light and reducing the roar of the city to a distant murmur. The car edged forward between sleek limousines that lined the kerbsides before finally coming to a halt in front of a pair of black iron gates. When they swung open, as if propelled by unseen hands, the car passed through and Holly caught sight of a white-haired old woman, the concierge, at the window of her lodge, nodding to the chauffeur whose gloved hand rose to acknowledge her greeting. In the centre of the courtyard a fountain was playing gently in the afternoon sunshine, its warm golden stone ringed by a bed of early red geraniums. The car circled it slowly, its tyres crunching on the gravel, and drew up before a flight of stone steps that led to an imposing entrance.

Leaving Henri to deal with their luggage, Holly followed Arlette inside the building and across the marble floor of the lobby towards the lift. Arlette leaned heavily on the brass button beside the Art Nouveau latticework of its doors.

"Ma chère Holly, my feet are – how you English say – killing me dead. Londres and back in only four days – never again! Jamais! Jamais!" Though she loved speaking English Arlette's quick brain and Latin temperament meant that her tongue could never keep pace with her thoughts and the result was usually an attractive mix of both languages.

The cage of the lift descended and they stepped inside. Arlette kicked off her stilettos and nestled her stockinged feet into the deep pile of the crimson carpet. The facetted mirrors set into the polished mahogany walls reflected their images as they ascended slowly. Not for the first time Holly thought how Arlette's flawless appearance belied her exhaustion. Her straight-backed figure was, as always, immaculate in a black Chanel tweed suit trimmed with matching braid. The cream bow of her crêpe de Chine blouse and the pearls at her neck superbly complemented her smooth olive skin. Yet Holly could see the weariness around her eyes and, when the lift reached the fifth floor, she quickly delved into her shoulder bag to find her own door key.

Inside the spacious apartment they parted, Arlette going to her study to telephone her editor-in-chief and Holly retiring to her own room. Tiny and tucked away in the attic, it could only be reached by a narrow back staircase. Originally it had been part of the servants' quarters – in fact the cook, Madame Tourbie, had the adjoining one – and Holly loved it. It was sparsely furnished with a cast-iron bedstead, a bedside table, a chest of drawers with an antique washstand, a wooden desk, one chair and a small wardrobe. There was a single mansard window below which the city of Paris lay spread out before her, stretching into the distance to the basilica of the Sacré-Cœur, perched like an iced wedding-cake on the hill of Montmartre.

Holly opened the casement, pushed back the shutters and leaned out. The hum of the city rose to greet her. Despite her tiredness she lingered there, once more recalling the day of her arrival when she had stood at the same spot, praying that she had made the right decision, knowing that for the months to come this strange house in this unknown city was to be her home. There had been a gentle tap on her door, the knob had turned slowly and an elfin face had peeped round it.

"Bonjour mademoiselle. Je suis Virginie. Vous avez fait un bon voyage?" Arlette's daughter had been five years old, a child with perfect manners, blessed with inborn grace and natural beauty, with huge dark eyes and long black hair that tumbled in ringlets onto her white organdie dress. She had been born to Arlette and her husband Henri after ten childless years of marriage and they adored her.

Holly turned abruptly from the window at the pain of the memory. Only four months later Virginie and her father had been killed when the small plane he was flying back from a visit to his parents in Belgium had crashed outside Paris in the woods near

Compiègne. Poor, poor Arlette. Since then she had been alone in her vast apartment with her cook, maid, chauffeur and Holly, the au pair who had suddenly lost her raison d'être. Arlette had refused to hear that Holly should look for another position. Plunging herself into her work as a fashion editor, she had begged Holly to stay on as her personal assistant and companion, perhaps in the desperate hope that this young woman's presence might bring her some slight consolation for the loss of the daughter whom she would never see grow up.

At first Holly's duties had mainly consisted of taking telephone messages or running errands, but as her command of the language and, with it, her self-confidence grew, she had found herself increasingly caught up in Arlette's work. This involved commissioning fashion articles, arranging photo shoots and reviewing the twice-yearly collections of the great couturiers. As the months passed, Arlette had begun to notice Holly's intuitive sense of style and colour. When her fortieth birthday made her painfully aware that she was growing older, she was glad to take Holly on assignments, knowing that she could rely on her taste and her opinions to coincide with those of the magazine's younger readers.

Holly shut the window with a bang, as if in doing so she could shut the painful memories out. Before dinner she would have time to complete the rough sketches she had made in London. She should begin now, while the impressions were fresh in her mind. Crossing to her desk, she carefully placed her sewing-machine on the floor and bundled a heap of soft grey flannel into a carrier bag to make space. The machine had belonged to her mother. It was heavy and awkward to carry, but it was one of the few possessions she had brought from England and she could never have parted with it.

Quickly recognizing the total unsuitability of her English wardrobe for her new life, Holly had resisted the temptation to replace it with cheap fashions from the Parisian chain stores. Instead she had studied the photographs in Arlette's magazines. Sitting in a pavement café making a cup of coffee last as long as possible, she had spent hours watching the Parisiennes passing by. She had noted the superb fabrics and excellent cut of their clothes, the basic colours which they seemed to prefer and the importance of the accessories they chose. Slowly she had begun to understand that their world-renowned chic lay in their understatement, combined with an insistence on quality. Their clothes never dominated the wearer, but instead underlined her personality and style. In that way, she realized, a well-dressed woman became a beautiful woman, not just a woman wearing beautiful clothes.

After a while Holly had ventured to buy fabrics herself, searching for remnants of exquisite materials at bargain prices. Often she was lucky. Arlette helped her with suggestions but she always cut the patterns herself. A piece of cream silk became a blouse, a length of chocolate tweed a fitted jacket with leather buttons, three metres of russet wool a skirt with matching waistcoat, and the grey flannel on the floor would eventually become a trouser suit. Arlette's critical eye appraised Holly, though she said little, wanting to give her time to find her own way rather than impose ideas on her, but she was pleased with the way Holly's style and taste were developing.

Like so many of the French, Arlette loved to discuss, and in the evenings, over a glass of wine, she and Holly would sit and talk, not only on topics connected with fashion and journalism but also about politics and history, music and literature, art and the theatre. Their conversations often lasted far into the night. Holly knew that she had much to learn but was not afraid to advance her own opinions. Yet their discussions never touched their personal lives. She sensed that Arlette, like herself, could not bear to reveal the pain that lay deep within her and each respected the other too much to probe into the past. Both had suffered greatly, but the time for healing had not yet come.

Darkness fell as she worked to complete her sketches, carefully adding a line or a touch of shading to achieve the effect she wished to create. Leaning back at last and stretching her arms over her head in satisfaction, she heard the distant chimes of the clock in the hallway downstairs striking eight. She had been so engrossed she had not noticed that several hours had passed. She put her charcoal and pencils away quickly. Her tiredness had vanished and a pleasant sense of anticipation filled her at the thought of the evening ahead.

As in most Parisian households, dinner was seldom served before nine, but when guests were invited, Arlette liked everyone to assemble earlier in the salon for aperitifs. Holly never knew in advance who would be present. Often other journalists were there, editors, writers or photographers, occasionally diplomats or businessmen, some of whom had been friends or partners of Arlette's husband. Sometimes Holly found herself seated next to well-known actors, painters or musicians; sometimes young, unknown artists were invited, in which case she could never be sure whether Arlette wanted to further their careers or just give them a good meal. The food was lavish. Five courses were de rigueur, as if Madame Tourbie, compensating for the fact that breakfast was served in the bedrooms and lunch, if at all, was taken in town, put all her efforts into one sumptuous meal in order to justify her presence in the household.

Holly soaked luxuriously in the huge tub in the marble bathroom on the floor below before returning to her room, wrapped in one of Arlette's bathrobes. She vigorously towelled her hair dry then chose a simple dress of cream georgette from her wardrobe. She had made it herself and slipped it over her head, enjoying the coolness of the smooth fabric against her body. Arlette had been right, she thought, to advise her against black at her age. The soft warm tone complemented the bloom of her skin. Knowing how the candlelight which Arlette loved, while flattering the contours of her face, would drain the colour from it, she added a blush of rouge under her cheekbones and painted her lips in a dusky shade of rose. She brushed a hint of ivory shadow on her eyelids and applied two coats of mascara to her lashes. After slipping on a pair of gold evening sandals, a

Christmas present from Arlette, she checked her reflection in the long mirror inside her wardrobe before making her way down the back stairs to the floor below.

Raised male voices greeted her as she passed from the hall through the double doors that stood open, leading to the salon. Two men, their backs towards her, were in lively dispute. Comte Maurice de Villiers she recognized at once. Since the death of Arlette's husband the distinguished private banker had done everything within his power to help the widow of his former business partner and closest friend. He not only managed her financial interests but also advised her in all important matters. A week rarely passed without his visiting them and they were occasionally seen together at the opera or the theatre. Although Parisian society had begun to link the name of the solicitous middle-aged bachelor with that of his attractive companion, Holly sensed that Arlette's deep feelings of affection and gratitude towards him could not overcome the grief that remained locked in her heart.

They were speaking in French and it was the voice of the other, younger man which caught her ears as she approached the gilded drinks trolley where Arlette, elegant in a black Givenchy cocktail dress, was mixing martinis.

"Ma chère tante, I'm delighted you found your trip to London so productive. The English designers have ideas, yes, but how do they show their clothes? And who can wear them there? The best English women I have met all moved as if they were showing off a horse in the enclosure before a race, rather than showing clothes. The worst ones moved like horses themselves – and looked like them too!"

The tinkling sound as Arlette dropped a cube of ice from her silver tongs into a crystal tumbler broke the ensuing silence. She raised her eyes to Holly, causing the speaker to turn. His glance fell on her. Arlette smiled coolly at her guest, the diamond rings on her outstretched hand glittering in the dancing firelight as she handed Holly an aperitif.

"I think you have not met before. Holly, may I introduce

my nephew, Julien de Mervais? He has just returned from Singapore where he has been working for the last three years. Julien, this is Holly Barton, my personal assistant. From England," she added with mischievous emphasis.

Centuries of good breeding manifested themselves in the young Frenchman's face as he covered his embarrassment by bending swiftly over Holly's hand and raising it to his lips.

"Mademoiselle, je suis désolé." With the apology his eyes rose to meet hers. "Please allow me to reconsider my opinions," he added in perfect English with a slight French accent tinged with American.

Holly accepted her drink but had barely time to take more than a few sips before Arlette announced, "My dears, let us not keep Madame Tourbie waiting. I know she has been busy all day and I would not care to face her anger if we should allow her soufflé to collapse."

Amid the laughter that greeted these words, Maurice de Villiers offered Arlette his arm and, with Holly and Julien following, they passed through a further set of doors into the dining room.

The Louis Seize table was set for four. The Bohemian chandelier hung low, its candlelight gleaming softly on the glossy mahogany before fading away into the shadows of the deep velvet drapes at the windows. The table, as always, had a lush centrepiece of flowers; cream narcissi, white lilies and early mimosa from Provence echoed the richness of the green and gold Sèvres dinner service, the heavy silver cutlery, the ivory damask napkins and the clusters of crystal wine glasses at each place setting.

Holly paused while Julien drew back her chair for her, and another scene rose before her eyes: a farmhouse kitchen, a scrubbed table, simple blue and white china and a golden shepherd's pie. She took her seat thoughtfully, raising her gaze some moments later to see Julien, seated opposite her, his dark eyes staring intently into her own. She looked down quickly, pretending to concentrate on shaking out her napkin, but her heart was beating faster. No one had looked at her like that since . . . At once she pushed the thought to the back of her mind. She must return to the present. Julien's attention was no doubt simply an attempt to make up for his previous rudeness.

Faced with the serious business of dining, the guests applied themselves to the food. Arlette ate little, as ever, for fear of losing her figure, picking only tiny morsels from her plate. Holly loved the French cuisine and, not yet having reason to fear its consequences, enjoyed the meal. The mousse of asparagus soufflé was delicious, the sole in tarragon and lemon sauce exquisite, and the Châteaubriand rich and succulent. White wines of the Loire gave way to deep red Bordeaux. In keeping with the tradition of their country, her table companions did not hide their pleasure. Each dish was analyzed, praised on its merits, comparisons were drawn, culinary memories revived, recipes quoted and restaurant recommendations exchanged. Unable to add more than her simple appreciation, Holly took little part in the conversation that flew back and forth.

Throughout the entire meal she was constantly aware of the eyes opposite her, disconcerting, dancing with amusement at her obvious unease. She felt them appraising her hair, her face, her shoulders and the line of her breasts beneath the thin fabric of her dress. To challenge him she raised her gaze to meet his, but far from being embarrassed by the confrontation, he smiled slowly, his eyes slanting upwards over the smooth tanned skin of his high cheekbones, his lips parting to reveal even white teeth. He touched his mouth with his napkin then raised his goblet of claret, holding it almost at arm's length, seeming to study its rich colour but in fact looking at her through the ruby depths.

After the dishes of the main course had been removed and a sumptuous selection of cheeses placed before them, conversation turned to the subjects of art and music. Arlette and her husband had been patrons of the arts and avid theatre-goers, rarely missing a production at the Comédie Française, the opera or any of the other major Parisian stages. Arlette had recently resumed the habit, Maurice de Villiers acting as a more than willing escort. As the latest plays were reviewed, interpreted and criticized, Julien revealed himself to be a connoisseur of the Parisian cultural scene. Holly noted how intently Arlette listened to his opinions and how Maurice seized on the points he made and expanded them for further discussion.

As the dinner drew to a close, culminating in a magnificent Gâteau St. Honoré as dessert, the talk turned to a coming festival of the works of Verdi, which would be the highlight of the season at the Opéra.

"Perhaps you know *La Traviata*, ma chère?" Arlette was gently trying to draw Holly into their conversation. "The opera is based on the novel by Dumas, the tragic story of the courtesan, Marguerite Gautier, who was known as the Lady of the Camellias. She dies of consumption in the end. It's my own particular favourite."

"Yes." Holly spoke shyly, more to Arlette than to the others at the table. "My mother . . . " She paused, and with a barely discernible effort steadied her voice. "My mother had some records of Verdi's operas and we used to listen to them on winter evenings. She loved *La Traviata*." Julien's dark eyes never left her face as she spoke. The contours of his face seemed to soften in the flickering candlelight.

"Then be my guests, my dears!" Maurice suddenly broke the silence that followed her words. "I invite you all to be my guests at the première. I shall take a box at the Opéra . . ."

Arlette's silvery laughter interrupted him. "Mon cher Maurice, even you cannot get tickets for an event like that! Le Tout-Paris will be there! The performance has been sold out for months – ah, c'est impossible!" She shrugged her shoulders expressively.

"You will see, ma chère Arlette. Wait and see. . . "

Out of respect for Arlette's tiring day the evening did not end late. After coffee the two visitors took their leave, Maurice with sincere promises to procure the promised tickets, Julien with elegant words of thanks and kisses for his aunt. Once again he raised Holly's hand to his lips, and only she was aware that he held it there for a fraction longer than etiquette demanded.

Alone in her room at last, Holly slipped between the cool linen sheets, yet despite her exhaustion, a kaleidoscope of memories was spinning in her brain. Grey eyes that melted with her own. Fair curly hair that she once longed to reach out and touch. Words of love drowned in the wind howling down from the moors, and the roaring waves of the sea.

Dawn was breaking over Paris when at last she drifted into an uneasy sleep that would carry her away, far away to another time, another place where it had all begun . . .

TWO

North Yorkshire, December 1962

. . . The rough voice with its soft Yorkshire vowels is kind, and a broad, red-veined face beams at her. "I'll be off now, lass. Put the figures on my desk and lock up before you go."

"Sure, Mr Johnson. See you tomorrow."

The door closes behind him and the smell of petrol mingles with cigarette smoke as it drifts into the room. Huge wet snowflakes are falling softly past the window. Holly watches as the portly figure of her employer in his heavy overcoat disappears into the darkness outside. The heat from the two-bar gas-fire in the tiny office makes it hard to concentrate. She heaves a deep sigh and the harsh neon lighting that shines on her dark hair catches a sudden glint of auburn as she moves to cup her chin in her hand. The fine arches of her brows are drawn and her teeth bite into her red lower lip as she chews the end of her biro. The long columns of figures seem to taunt her mockingly, teasing her into making a mistake.

Yet she knows she should be grateful for this job. Her father was a simple hill farmer who left school at fourteen. When years of toil, sheep-farming in all weathers on the bleak windswept North Yorkshire moors, led to his early death, Holly and Elizabeth, her mother, were left alone at Black Ridge Farm in the rambling nineteenth-century farmhouse. The sheep and the land have long since been sold off. Elizabeth earns what she can by taking in sewing and dress-making, but money is always scarce and work hard to come by in the little market-town. Alan Johnson, the owner of three filling-stations, is one of the wealthiest men in the dale and one of the nicest too. Like most of the close-knit community of Ainsley, he knew of their plight and, when Holly left school that summer, told her he needed 'someone for the office'. At the time it seemed like a heaven-sent opportunity for her to boost their meagre income.

Holly stares at the figures that the pump attendant has scrawled on a scrap of paper. She has to check them against the till roll, add up the total sales of petrol for the day, subtract them from the figures of the last delivery and calculate the following week's orders. She starts to list the sums carefully, but her hand soon strays to the margin which she begins to illustrate with a winding garland of hedgerow flowers, bees and butterflies. Drawing is her greatest love, painting too, but it is her pencil that can transport her away from the stuffy office with its dingy filing cabinets and the thumbed calendars on the walls. Her imagination is overflowing with impressions of the countryside she loves: sturdy bell heather quivering under the first winter snow, pale primroses sparkling with crystal drops of spring dew, delicate dog-roses slumbering to the murmur of summer bees. Her sketchbook portrays momentary glimpses, seen through the eye of a born naturalist and created by the hand of an intuitive artist.

She forces herself to return to the figures on the desk and makes a final determined effort to concentrate. The language of mathematics means nothing to her, unlike French which has a flow and musicality that appeals to her artistic nature. Her French teacher at school has suggested she should study the language at university, but Holly knows that if she could ever afford to study, her future would lie in some form of art, perhaps design or illustration, a dream that is about as likely as a flight to the moon.

When she has at last drawn a double line under the total, she leans back in her chair frowning slightly. It is probably all wrong, she thinks, but Dorothy will check everything in the morning.

Dorothy is Mr Johnson's secretary, a proper secretary who has learnt shorthand and typing. Dorothy is everything that Holly is not, over twenty-one, poised and very self-assured in her Jackie Kennedy-style sheath dresses and pearly white stilettos. She has a lover, a married man, and, after several glasses of

Babycham on her birthday, confided to Holly that she had been abroad with him on an illicit holiday. Holly must have looked surprised because Dorothy laughed and said that it was 1962, not the fifties, but added that she had put a wedding ring on her finger all the same. When Holly asked her in a whisper whether the fear of getting pregnant had not spoilt the trip, Dorothy hinted darkly that there were 'ways and means' to avoid that, but frustratingly did not go into detail.

A tap on the window breaks into Holly's thoughts. In the darkness outside she makes out a muffled figure covered in snowflakes, leaning against a bicycle. She quickly puts the list of figures on her employer's desk, pulls on her duffle coat, locks the office and goes out to join her dearest friend. Florence Westbury is the daughter of the local GP and they have been inseparable since their first day at school – inseparable until three months ago when Flo went to study at a teacher-training college in York. Left behind in the dale, Holly did not know which was greater – her sadness at missing her friend, or her envy.

"How are you enjoying your vacation?" Holly hugs her friend.

"What vacation?" Flo groans in mock despair. "You should see the list of books I've got to get through before January! At this rate I'll be reading them on Christmas Day!"

They get on their bicycles and pedal up the steep road leading out of town. In the darkness a bitterly cold wind is sweeping down from the moors, tearing at their woollen hats and snapping at the hems of their coats. Eventually they stop in front of the Westburys' house, a plain but imposing Georgian residence in Yorkshire stone. Flo gets off her bike. "Are you coming carol-singing tonight?" she asks, panting slightly.

"What? Carol-singing?" Holly looks at her friend in amusement. "You don't mean that, do you? We haven't sung any carols since we were at school!"

"Come on," Flo urges. "It'll be fun, and it's for a good cause. We're collecting for the new wing at the hospital."

"Why will it be fun?" Holly does not sound convinced.

"Well, Dave's going – we're taking his car – and Jane. And I think Mike's coming along as well," she adds with an air of nonchalance.

"Ah, I see!" Holly smiles knowingly at her friend. She has long guessed that Flo is in love with Mike.

"You don't see anything at all!" Flo looks indignant. "Anyway, it'll be a great chance for us all to meet up again, now everyone's gone away to college – " She stops and her hand flies to her mouth. "Oh I'm sorry, Holly! I shouldn't have said that!"

"It's alright." Holly grins ruefully. "I'd love to go with you but I think I should stay in and help Mum. Georgina Ranleigh at the Hall has asked her to make a dress from some material she's got and Mum wants me to cut it out for her."

"I wish you could design something for me," Flo sighs wistfully. "I bet one of your creations would make even me look slim." She looks down at her well-rounded hips which her heavy gabardine coat does nothing to hide, before glancing at Holly's slim figure.

"You're fine the way you are. I wouldn't want you any different. But just you wait." Holly's brown eyes dance. "When I get my own label you can be sure that one of the designs in my first collection will be especially for you!"

Laughing, they part and Holly pedals on up the hill leading out to the head of the dale. She pulls off her cap and her long hair swirls behind her in the wind.

Flurries of snow are starting to fall again as she opens the gate to Black Ridge Farm and enters the yard. When she wheels her bike into the empty stable, her eye falls on the row of dusty harnesses and reins, festooned with cobwebs, hanging along the wall. As a child, she had her own pony but nowadays there is scarcely enough money to feed her mother and herself. There is no question of keeping any animals. She can remember her eighth birthday when the pony arrived, how she clung to the saddle, shrieking with joy as her father ran beside her, one hand holding the bridle, the other firmly grasping the back of her dungarees. Soon afterwards he died, killed by a bout of pneumonia after a winter's night spent on the moors, searching for lost sheep buried in drifts of snow. It is strange, she thinks, how she can remember her first ride so clearly and yet she can hardly recall his face. Sometimes she even wonders whether her recollections of him are memories at all and not simply inspired by the photo of the young man with the shy smile, which her mother so cherishes.

As she enters the farmhouse kitchen, Elizabeth Barton quickly places a log on the fire in the range, but Holly notices the coldness of the room where her mother has been working. A large heap of unfinished sewing is lying on the scrubbed wooden table. Elizabeth at once bundles it aside and begins laying two places for their evening meal. Like most Yorkshire folk of her age she does not hold with kissing or touching in greeting.

"Come on in, love. You look right frozen. Shepherd's pie for tea," she says warmly and raises one thin arm to take down two worn blue and white plates from the dresser.

Holly sits down at the table and, as she does every weekday, begins to entertain her mother with stories of happenings at the office. She always elaborates on any funny incident she can remember, conscious of the fact that, apart from visits to clients for whom she sews, and a weekly trip to the market, Elizabeth Barton has no contact with the world beyond the farmhouse. Dark-haired, slender and delicately-boned, she is quite unlike the other local farmers' wives. Her white, almost translucent skin and the dark green of her eyes, like deep pools of water in a woodland glade, give her a fragile beauty which the harsh climate of the moors has enhanced rather than dispelled. A judge's daughter, she married against her parents' wishes. Perhaps that is why she has never seemed part of country life.

Holly watches as her mother pulls an oven cloth from the airer strung high above her head, carefully opens the heavy iron door of the kitchen range and takes out a bubbling, golden-brown shepherd's pie. Its delicious smell fills the room. Suppressing a slight cough, she places the dish on the table.

"Mum, have you been to see Dr Westbury yet? You've had that cough for ages."

"Just don't you worry. I'll be fine," her mother murmurs. "I heard at the market that there'll be carol-singing this evening. Why don't you go along? See your friends again now they're all back home for Christmas."

Holly sees through her mother's attempt to distract her attention from her personal problems. "I thought I'd stay in and cut out Georgina Ranleigh's dress."

"There's no hurry, love, I've still got the smocking to do on the christening robe for the vicar's new baby. You go along. You should be out with other young folks, not stuck in here with me every evening."

Holly thinks for a moment. "Alright, Mum," she says at last. "But only if you promise me you'll see Dr Westbury in the morning." Elizabeth nods her assent, saying nothing, and Holly knows that, for tonight at least, the matter has been brought to a close.

It is nearly seven o'clock when she reaches the Market Cross in the High Street where the carol-singers have arranged to meet. Flo's face lights up when she sees Holly arriving on her bicycle and her other friends greet her cheerfully. Holly scrambles into the back of Dave's old Morris Minor while Flo gets into the passenger seat. Squashed between Mike and Dave's sister, Jane, Holly listens to the evening's itinerary.

"We're heading for the Hall first," Dave announces, revving the engine vigorously and leaning against the car door as if to compensate for the gravitational pull as they round a corner at breakneck speed. "Might as well start where the pickings are richest. The Ranleighs should cough up ten shillings for a good cause."

Within minutes they have left the town behind and turned from a wooded country lane into a long winding drive. The headlamps of the car spill through the darkness, revealing dense rhododendron bushes on either side. The stillness awes them into silence and Dave even slows the car to walking pace. Presently the drive opens out to reveal a Jacobean manor house surrounded by huge fir trees. The wind moans through their tossing branches and clouds race across the pale moon. The red-brick, ivy-clung walls seem overpowering, stretching up to tall chimneys that loom against the dark sky. The leaded windows are unlighted. Only a solitary lantern is swinging slightly in the porch, casting fitful shadows on the heavy wooden door.

Flo, practical as ever, has brought sheets of music which she hands round. Having grown up with the traditional Christmas carols, they are all long familiar with the tunes but far from certain when it comes to remembering the words. After a tremulous start their voices gather strength. Their surroundings are soon forgotten in the spell cast as a time-worn melody with its meaningful words unfolds. Holly's clear soprano rings out above the others' voices, leading them through the verses. When the last notes have died away, Dave grasps the great iron knocker. Within the house there is the sound of footsteps coming nearer and the bolts of the massive door are drawn back. As it swings open, light fills the porch and an elderly woman, dressed in grey, appears smiling on the threshold and invites them inside.

In silent procession they cross the entrance hall. A polished oak floor covered with worn Persian carpets, and high walls hung with antlers and other hunting trophies are fleeting impressions before a pair of double doors open to reveal a family sitting-room. Holly is instantly reminded of that magic moment when, as a child, she saw Flo's dolls-house for the first time and gazed inside. Now, as then, she is a spectator with no place in the scene that lies before her.

A huge inglenook fireplace filled with burning logs and surrounded by gleaming copper utensils of a bygone age dominates the room. The spines of leather-bound books lining the walls glow richly in the flickering firelight. Heavy, gold velvet curtains at the long windows blend with the warm red and orange hues of chintzes covering the sofa and armchairs grouped around the fire.

"Hello. Please come in. You must be frozen, it's so cold

outside. Do sit down and warm yourselves up. Would you like a drink?" A tall, slim young woman with fair hair that softly frames her heart-shaped face rises to greet them. Holly introduces her friends. Elizabeth Barton sewed for Georgina when she was a child and Holly can remember accompanying her mother to Ranleigh Hall on those occasions. She was the little girl in the worn clothes who stood awkwardly holding the pins whilst her mother knelt before this other, slightly older child, fitting a silk party frock, a gingham summer dress or a velvet-collared coat. Soon after, Georgina was whisked away to complete her education at a private school in the south of England. They met again only recently when Georgina drove over to Black Ridge Farm with some material that she wanted Elizabeth to make into an evening dress for her.

"Perhaps you'd rather have a cup of tea instead of sherry?" A voice breaks into her thoughts and Holly is embarrassed to realize that Georgina is asking her for the second time.

"No – thanks – sherry would be lovely," she manages to stammer in reply. Georgina's shining hair curves smoothly over her cheek as she bends to pour from the decanter. "She's so beautiful," Holly thinks, and a pang of envy shoots through her. She gazes intently at the amber liquid glowing in its crystal glass on the antique rosewood table. All this, such a home and beauty too . . . it does not seem fair somehow.

"And you, Mother?" It is only then that Holly becomes aware of Lady Marianne Ranleigh, a tiny figure hunched in a wheelchair beside the fire. Thin, with black hair drawn severely back from what was once a lovely face, she resembles a little bird. "I'm sure Mother would love to hear you sing again," Georgina says, handing her mother a cup of tea which she takes with such trembling hands that Dave rushes forward to help her place the delicate bone china on a pedestal table at her side.

While they sing once more, Holly's mind flies back to snippets of gossip she has heard in town . . ."Terrible accident . . . paralysed from the waist down . . . wheelchair for the rest of her life . . . that awful husband of hers . . ." She thinks gratefully of her own mother, so active, so untiring, and notices how Georgina turns the invalid round from the fireplace so that she can hear better, stirs her tea for her and helps her raise the cup to her lips.

Some minutes later when she has slipped a pound-note into their collecting box, Georgina leads them into the hall where they are handed their coats.

"Thanks so much for coming. You don't know how much this has meant to Mother. Since Father died she doesn't go out much and hardly ever gets to meet anyone at all." Her lips form a shy smile, but Holly sees the sadness in her eyes. When the door has closed behind them, she glances back towards the great house. It looks even more foreboding than before. She wonders what secrets it holds.

Sounds of the car door slamming and the engine springing into life interrupt Holly's reverie. She huddles down inside her coat for warmth, shivering slightly in the biting night air. Mike shifts his weight to give her more room and then gently, quite casually, raises his arm to place it round her shoulders. It is an almost brotherly gesture and she is uncertain how to react. She prays that Flo will not turn round and see.

It is at that moment, as they are turning out of the drive onto the main road again, that a low-slung red sports car suddenly appears from nowhere. Blinded by its headlights, Dave curses and tears at the steering wheel, almost catapulting them into the ditch by the roadside. Missing them by inches the MG swings into the drive, its tyres screeching, and roars off in the direction from which they themselves have just come. The whole incident has taken only seconds but it leaves Holly shaken and puzzled.

It seems that the quiet genteel household at the manor house is to receive a most unlikely visitor.

THREE

Paris, Spring 1967

Holly pulled herself onto one elbow, rubbing the sleep from her eyes. The memories fled like shadows, chased by the shafts of sunlight that patterned the bedroom floor.

"Bonjour, mademoiselle."

Marie, the maid, entered with a jug of hot water for the washstand, then returned only minutes later carrying a tray of black coffee, hot milk and freshly-baked croissants. She placed it on a small table beside the bed before opening the windows inwards and leaning out to bang back the shutters. The warmth and buzz of the city poured into the room. "Madame requests you to come to her as soon as possible."

Holly washed and breakfasted quickly, then pulled on a sweater and trousers – Arlette would never allow anyone under any circumstances to wear jeans under her roof – and ran lightly downstairs to what Arlette always referred to as her 'boudoir'. She knocked, and at the call of "Entrez!" went into the room to find Arlette sitting up in bed, her negligée round her shoulders, daintily dipping a croissant into a bowl of black coffee as she leafed through her correspondence. Torn envelopes, opened letters, cards, bills and brochures were spread over the apricot silk counterpane.

"Bonjour, ma chère," she greeted Holly. "Tu as déjeuné, non?" Hearing that Holly had already breakfasted, Arlette turned to business at once. "See what is here. Invitations for the collections. We must plan how to fit the most important shows in, and don't forget there are the Italian ones too."

The next two hours were spent comparing the times and locations of the shows given by the world's leading fashion houses: Dior, Chanel, Saint-Laurent, Lavin, Patou, Givenchy – the names alone were magic to Holly's ears. Eventually they had a tightly-packed schedule drawn up, spanning a period of three weeks and taking them from Paris to Milan and on to Rome. Matters would have been easier if they could have flown from one city to another, but since the tragic crash in which she had lost her husband and child, Arlette had never boarded a plane again.

"I know I can leave the travel arrangements to you, chérie," she concluded with a sigh of relief. She yawned and stretched out her arms cat-like, scattering the papers which drifted gently to the floor. "Oh, I nearly forgot to tell you. The Comte de Villiers has sent a note this morning to say that he has reserved a – how do you say? – a loge at the opera."

"A box?" Holly gasped. "You mean a box at the opera?" She asked again, feeling foolish at the sound of her own words.

"Mais oui. Of course. It is for the première of *La Traviata* in two weeks' time. I wonder how many strings he has pulled to arrange that? We shall be dining after the performance at Maxim's."

"But madame, I couldn't . . . I mean I can't possibly . . . I mean I haven't got . . ."

Arlette interrupted Holly's stammering with a smile. "Chérie, we are his guests and he has especially extended the invitation to include both you and Julien. You don't want to disappoint him, do you?"

Holly only managed to gulp and shake her head in reply.

"And as for the matter of a gown for you, don't worry about that. I will borrow a little something from one of the ateliers. There are several designers I can think of who owe me a favour. Ça va sans dire. And now, vite, vite! Run along and make those travel arrangements to Italy for us."

Holly went along the corridor to Arlette's study. She sat down at the Directoire desk and opened its scroll top. Stretching out her hand to pick up the telephone receiver, her eye fell on Arlette's appointments diary which lay open in front of her. It was March 10th, the anniversary of the day she had left England to come to France two years ago. Had she made the right decision? If she had stayed in England, where would she have been now? What would her life have been like? She would never know.

She pushed those thoughts aside. Lifting the phone she began to dial the number of Arlette's favourite hotel in Milan. The trip she was about to book was a journey into the future, not into the past.

The days that followed seemed to pass in a dream. As fashion editor of *Mode et Beauté*, Arlette attended the shows of the coming autumn-winter collections of all the great couturiers and Holly felt thrilled and privileged to accompany her. But despite their glamorous invitation cards, they had to struggle with hundreds of other journalists for admittance to the great couture houses. Once inside, Arlette could claim a seat, though only the very rich or very famous could expect to be in the front row; Holly had to stand at the back, craning her neck to watch some of the world's most beautiful women take the catwalks in some of the world's most gorgeous clothes. All the while she was sketching hastily, scribbling notes, jotting down details, recording impressions. It was a fight for survival, jostling for position in hot, overcrowded rooms, everyone wanting to be the first to capture the next season's trends and publish them to the world. It was a fight that left them both exhausted by the end of each day.

Holly was aware that she was learning all the time. Like a sponge she was absorbing all she could about fashion, with Arlette as a more than willing and able teacher.

"Et bien, ma chère Holly, what do you think of what you have seen this morning?" Arlette always asked her opinion first after each show. Holly believed that, in doing so, Arlette wanted to avoid imposing her own ideas on her young protégée; it never entered her mind that the older woman actually valued the fresh approach of an open-minded twenty- two-year old. They had just left the Courrèges show and were sitting outdoors in a restaurant under the arcade of the Place des Vosges, Arlette having declared herself incapable of walking another step without lunch.

Holly thought for a moment before replying. "Exciting, shocking, innovative, futuristic, space-hits-fashion . . . those mini-dresses and coats with hats like helmets and the thick tights and flat boots, all in white and silver – the models looked like spacemen, didn't they?"

Arlette shook open her napkin as their salads arrived. "Well, the Russians put a man in space six years ago and they say that the Americans are planning to land on the moon one day, so it's more reality than future. I think it's a look we'll be seeing on the high street soon. Did you notice how Courrèges always leaves about three centimetres between the garment and the body? That's why his clothes always look so comfortable. Like sportswear." She laughed. "You know, one day I fear people will start wearing sports clothes all the time! T-shirts to the office and anoraks in town! Imagine! Quelle horreur!" She gave a mock shudder and rearranged the Hermès silk scarf at her neck.

Encouraged, Holly ventured further. "Courrèges' style reminds me of Mary Quant in a way. You know, those baby- doll dresses and coats, geometric hairstyles and bobs we saw in London."

"How clever of you to notice." Arlette smiled at her. "Nobody is really in agreement about where the mini was invented – in London or Paris – but I tend to think it was in boutiques like Mary Quant's, or Biba on the Kings Road, followed by Carnaby Street. That's where they started to make inexpensive clothes for girls who didn't want to wear the same as their mothers were wearing."

"Well, the mothers are copying their daughters now, aren't they!"

"They certainly are," Arlette agreed. "Especially now that Paris has taken over and perfected the look with beautifully-cut clothes in gorgeous materials – such lovely soft wools and cashmeres."

"As long as you don't count Paco Rabanne," Holly countered. "What did you think of those dresses made of squares of metal fastened together with strips of leather? How on earth can you sit down in anything like that?"

Arlette laughed. "I don't think you're meant to! Rabanne is just trying to provoke us and open our eyes. I'm sure the next decades will see clothes made of materials nobody has even heard of today."

Holly sipped her Perrier thoughtfully. "Fashion changes so fast, doesn't it, madame?"

Arlette's dark eyes glowed. "That's what I love about this business. It never stands still! Mon Dieu, I remember the fashions in the fifties. Dior's New Look came out when I was a young fashion journalist just starting out. It seemed so sensationally avant-garde, pure glamour after the austerity of the war years! And how do we see Dior's New Look nowadays? Pouf!" She shrugged expressively. "Women with sharp pointed bosoms and nipped-in waists over huge skirts, all stiff and unnatural with their permed hair and pouting red lips! Today we have the exact opposite – the Lolita look with big smudgy eyes, pale face, Vidal Sassoon haircut, short dress, long legs – but you know, my dear, in another five years that will be passé, too! As you said, fashion changes very fast."

"Weren't models called mannequins in those days?"

"Yes, they were, but you can't really compare them. The mannequins were almost plump by today's standards, and I don't mean Twiggy – you know I think that girl's so thin she should be in hospital! – I mean compared to the lovely models we have today like Jean Shrimpton or Penelope Tree."

A dreamy look came into Holly's eyes. "Fabulous . . . and Veruschka – she's my favourite."

"They move so beautifully now. The mannequins used to pose. Today we have action on the catwalk but that's because lots of women are on the move as well – they don't just stay at home waiting for their husbands any more – so the clothes they wear have to move with them!" She caught the waiter's eye and called for the bill. "And speaking of moving, ma chère, it's time for us to move too if we don't want to miss Saint-Laurent. Now that's a show that will be much more to my taste. I'm sure there won't be a spaceman in sight!"

Arlette was not to be disappointed. Holly stared open-mouthed in delight and admiration as the models took the catwalk. Short coats and dresses with geometric designs in red, blue, green and yellow, outlined with black on white backgrounds, paid homage to op art. Arlette told her later that the young designer had been influenced by his friend Andy Warhol and the works of Picasso, Matisse and Mondrian, but Holly could see for herself how the bold colours matched the simple, clean lines.

They were succeeded by an African-inspired theme, a medley of eminently wearable tunics, pants, skirts and dresses in rich creams, oranges and browns including a belted safari jacket which was greeted with such tumultuous applause that it was clear that every woman in the room would have given a month's wages to possess it. Holly could see Diana Vreeland, chief editor of *Vogue*, scribbling furiously in her notebook.

Jewel-coloured evening gowns in richly embroidered silks and satins, velvets and brocades followed; each one would make its fortunate wearer feel like royalty. When Holly thought that nothing could surpass what she had just seen, Veruschka von Lehndorff appeared, tall, willowy and feline in a sensational black evening suit. This superbly feminine version of the male garment with nothing but bare tanned skin underneath drew standing ovations. Holly noticed Cathérine Deneuve in the front row looking enchanted. Such elegance merging with pure sex appeal might have been designed with the beautiful young actress in mind.

At the end of the show, Saint-Laurent himself was dragged protesting onto the catwalk. Painfully thin and shy, he looked more like an overgrown schoolboy than a great couturier. Holly was on her feet with the rest, clapping and cheering until her hands hurt and her ears rang.

In the car returning home, Arlette could not cease praising the young designer. "So talented, so brilliant! Do you know, ma chère, he started with Dior but after three years they quarrelled and he left to create his own house. And now he has a new idea, it's called prêt-à-porter – how do you say – 'ready to wear'? The French sounds so much better, n'est-ce pas? He thinks that the days of the great maisons de couture are over. Perhaps he is right. How many women can afford to pay for suits and gowns that have been custom-made these days? And surely it is not only the rich who have the right to be elegant?"

Holly sighed. "I thought that trouser suit he showed was sensational – masculine, but at the same time feminine, even erotic. I'm sure any woman would feel supremely self-confident wearing it."

"It's amazing, isn't it, how he has achieved one look for daytime and another for evening wear. It's as if a woman has to compete with men during the day – without losing her femininity of course – but after dark she can revert to being solely a woman again." Arlette chattered on enthusiastically but Holly had fallen silent. She had loved the collections. She had been enthralled, inspired, at times even shocked by what she had seen. And the best had come last.

When their limousine drew up in front of the apartment, Holly went to her room. Her body told her that she should rest, but her mind was caught up in a ceaseless whirl of activity. She sat down at her desk, pulling her sketchbook out of her shoulder bag, and spread the drawings she had made in front of her. Even without the notes she had taken she knew at once which show each referred to, just as she had known instinctively which clothes to sketch, which lines to emphasize and what to ignore. She had intuitively recognized the trends, almost as if she could read each designer's handwriting. But had she managed to transfer that knowledge onto paper? Would her work succeed in putting across the great designers' ideas to someone who had not been to the shows? She could only hope so.

She set the papers aside. Arlette had made it clear that, for her, this day's work was over, that she wanted nothing more than a relaxing hot bath and hoped that Holly would join her for a dinner à deux at eight in the evening. Holly showered and changed into a crisp white shirt and a pair of tailored black trousers, knowing that even a simple meal alone with Arlette did not mean that she could be too casually dressed.

When she entered the salon, Holly saw that two places had been set at a small table in front of the fire. The warmth of the spring day had gone and darkness was falling beyond the deep drapes at the windows. Candles on the mantelpiece and logs burning in the marble fireplace bathed the room in a soft glow. Dispensing with the usual cocktails, Arlette poured them both a glass of white wine which Holly gratefully accepted. Leaning back into the soft cushions of the velvet sofa, she stretched out her legs, feeling more comfortable than she had all day.

Madame Tourbie served a light dish of grilled fish with fresh Mediterranean vegetables. Holly found she was surprisingly hungry and ate with enjoyment. It was only after a while that she noticed Arlette had barely touched her food.

"Aren't you feeling well, madame?"

"I'm fine, ma chère." Arlette put down her knife and fork. Her face took on a serious expression. "My dear, there is something we should talk about."

Holly froze. Had she done something wrong? Some dreadful breach of etiquette? Something she had said that had offended someone? Her French was adequate but by no means perfect.

"I think we should discuss your future, Holly."

Holly's stomach muscles contracted. She forced herself to swallow. The delicious food had taken on a bitter taste. Was her work not good enough? Was her presence in the apartment disturbing Arlette? Surely her life in Paris could not be coming to an end? It was like being on an island, a magical tropical island where she was safe from storms and dangers. Was she about to lose her sanctuary?

Seeing Holly's stricken look, Arlette leaned across the table and patted her hand. As she did so, Holly realized that, apart from perfunctory greetings and goodbyes when they embraced, kissing in the French manner, this was the first time that Arlette had actually touched her. Was she trying to prepare her for bad news?

"You have been such a valuable assistant to me over the past two years," Arlette began slowly, "but I feel that the time has come for . . . "

"Please, madame. Don't send me away! Tell me what I've done wrong. I'll move out, if you like, I'll work for less money, anything you want, if only you don't . . . "

Arlette stared at Holly in amazement before breaking into a peal of laughter. "My dear, what makes you think I am not satisfied with your work? Do you even imagine that I'd want you to leave my home? Quelle idée absurde!" Shaking her head in amusement at the thought, she poured herself another glass of wine before she spoke again.

"I have been watching you, my dear, seeing how your work is developing. You have great talent." Holly opened her mouth to protest but Arlette silenced her with a raised hand. "Believe me, ma chère, I have been in the fashion business long enough to recognize talent when I see it. At first I wondered whether you might be suitable to apply for a position on the magazine . . . "

"But madame," Holly managed to break in at last, "I really love working as your personal assistant . . ."

"That may be so, but it's not what I meant. That isn't a proper job. Trotting around behind me all day – anyone could do that. How do you say in English – any dog can do that!"

"Dog?"

"Dogsbody! Now that is an expression I have never understood, but I suppose it is because the English all love dogs. No, I think you should concentrate on designing fashion yourself."

"Me? Design?" Holly eyes widened in amazement. "But I'm not trained. I mean, I've never studied properly. I haven't any real qualifications. I don't know enough about fashion."

"If that were true, my dear, I would not have taken you with me today, or any other day for that matter. There are enough people at the magazine who would give everything to go with me to the shows! Your understanding of fashion is intuitive, just as your talent for design is inborn. Of course you have a lot to learn and you will have to do so from the bottom, but I think you are willing and I will be here to help you."

"How, exactly?" Holly was incredulous but curious.

"As long as you wish you can go on working for me, but in the longer view you should look towards finding a place on the other side of the fashion business – not among those who report on fashion but among those who create it."

Holly's head was reeling.

"But how?" was all she managed to stammer again.

Arlette delicately lifted a sliver of fish on her fork to her mouth and chewed it thoughtfully before she spoke again.

"I'm not sure. But a chance will come, and when it does, I hope you will be willing to grasp it with both hands." She refilled Holly's glass, then raised her own. "To you, my dear."

Arlette's words echoed in Holly's brain as she sat at her window late that night. She had put into words what Holly herself had not dared to hope. Gazing out over the lights of the city, she knew beyond any shadow of doubt that her future lay in the world of fashion. But would she find her place there? The catwalk scenes from the shows flashed like coloured slides, clicking through her mind. Could she, Holly Barton from Yorkshire, in any way compete with what she had seen that day?

It was a dream. But was it an impossible dream? Wasn't a dream also a goal? Something you should not lose sight of? Something you would give up everything else to achieve? Her thoughts flew back in time and she wondered if she would ever forget where and when she had heard those words before . . .

FOUR

North Yorkshire, December 1962

. . . Inky black clouds race across the lowering sky, chasing their own shadows on the earth below as she battles with her easel. *Time to go*; the title of her painting is already in her mind. She longs to capture the moment when the wind rises to fever pitch, whipping and snapping the branches of the solitary trees on the moors, when patches of sunlight on the heather flee for safely into the folds of the dales, when heaven blackens and the menacing storm breaks forth to pour itself upon the waiting landscape. Grasping her flapping sketchbook with one hand, she adds several bold strokes of deep violet before heavy drops of rain start to descend with increasing force.

Quickly she closes her sketchbook and fastens the clasp of her paint box. Wet strands of her long dark hair are blowing into her eyes. She can feel the bitter wind cutting through her thin coat and the damp seeping through the soles of her shoes. A sudden tiredness overwhelms her. She has been so engrossed in her painting that she has lost all sense of time. She looks round in desperation. Where can she run for shelter?

The crags. The crags on the moor top where she went climbing with her father when she was a child cannot be far away. Panting hard she struggles forward over the clumps of heather, stumbling over the uneven ground, her easel clamped under one arm, her sketchbook clutched to her breast with the other. There is only one thought inside her head: she has to save this painting. It is far from complete, but this time she has achieved what has been eluding her for so long. She must not let it get spoilt by the driving rain, now rapidly turning into sleet.

Bent almost double, she fights her way up the hill. Her heart is pounding in her ears with the effort. When she feels her right foot slip and twist in a rut beneath her, a fierce pain shoots through her ankle and it is too late to stop herself from falling headlong into the heather. Her clothes are drenched with icy moorland water. The precious sketchbook is lying open on the ground beside her, its covers fluttering noisily in the wind as raindrops spatter on the delicate brushwork, the carefully chosen hues mingling and running in an ugly channel down the page into the sodden earth. Holly bends her head to the ground, her throat tightens and hot tears burn behind her eyes.

"Hey, what's the matter? Are you hurt?"

As if from a distance she hears a male voice. She raises her head slightly to see wet jeans over a pair of black boots. A border collie is poking its nose inquisitively into her face. Strong hands are grasping her, raising her none too gently to her feet. "You alright?"

"My ankle. Perhaps it's broken. I can't put any weight on it." She winces at the attempt. At the same moment she finds herself being lifted into the air.

"Put your arms round my neck and I'll try to carry you as far as the crags to get you out of the rain."

He sways under her weight, struggles to regain his balance, then carries her across the stretch of moorland dividing them from an outcrop of rocks that form a cave-like shelter, where he almost drops her onto the coarse dry grass.

"Whew, you're a lot heavier than you look!" he remarks ungallantly, panting with exertion. "Whatever are you doing up here anyway, lying around on the moors in the middle of winter? Playing Wuthering Heights?"

Holly pushes her wet hair out of her face and stares at her rescuer in astonishment. For once in her life she is at a loss for words. He is not the middle-aged farmer she imagined. A tousled mop of fair hair frames a lightly-tanned face and the grey eyes that meet hers crinkle in amusement. He looks to be in his early twenties and his thick navy sweater, now sodden with rain, reveals a slim athletic build. He is not one of the local men, she knows for certain. His features are finely-chiselled, like one of the

Greek statues in her art book. But what is a Greek god doing on a Yorkshire hillside?

Holly's sense of humour quickly overcomes her acute discomfort. "Sorry, Heathcliff. It won't happen again."

His eyes smile back at her. "What about that ankle?" he asks, kneeling down beside her. Holly moves her foot slightly, with a quick intake of breath as pain stabs through it.

"Let me have a look." Gently he eases off her boot and woollen sock. She quivers as he touches her bare skin. He bends her foot carefully, tracing the bones with long, tapering fingers. "I don't think it's broken," he finally announces, "but it's definitely a nasty sprain. Do you live near here?"

"Yes, at Black Ridge Farm," Holly murmurs, gazing at the head still bowed over her foot. The slight bronze stubble on his firm jawline dints to a tiny cleft on his chin. When his eyes rise and meet hers again, something inside her breast seems to lurch violently. The blood rushes to her face, making her cheeks burn. She thinks he must be able to hear her heart beating.

"I'll do my best to get you there but it's quite a way. I think we'd better wait till the rain stops." He sits down on the grass beside her. "Seriously, I really meant it when I asked what you were doing here. It's not the place for a girl to be on her own in December. I'm Nick, by the way," he adds, almost as an afterthought.

"Holly." She smiles back at him, despite the pain which has become a steady ache in her ankle. "I was painting – a water-colour, but at the moment there's more water than colour in my picture!" She shows him the ruined page of her sketchbook.

He does not laugh but studies her work intently. "It's very good. Or at least what's left of it is." He frowns when she tries to contradict. "No, honestly, I think it's great. You've managed to capture the atmosphere when a storm is just about to break on the moors." He hands the book back to her. "You've got terrific talent." He does not say the words casually, but sincerely.

This time she accepts the compliment. "Painting and sketching are what I enjoy most."

"Are you going to make a career out of it?"

Holly stares at him. They have met only moments ago and yet already she feels that he can read her innermost thoughts and secret dreams.

"I'd like to," she confesses, "but . . ." She cannot go on. How could her mother's tiny income ever stretch to supporting her at college?

"If that's your dream, you mustn't lose sight of it. You have to have a goal in life, something you would give up everything else to achieve. That's how much medicine means to me."

"You're studying to be a doctor?"

"Yes." He is pulling at a tuft of heather where they are sitting. "That's what I've wanted to do as long as I can remember."

"But that's great. It's far more important to be able to heal people and stop them suffering than to paint pictures or sketch things."

He suddenly turns to face her. "You must never think that!" He speaks quite fiercely. "Of course medicine is vital, but if there were no beautiful pictures, no good architecture, no lovely clothes or nice cars, no well-designed objects in our homes, I think we'd all suffer too."

"Are you nearly finished at university?" she ventures shyly.

"I have another couple of years to do before I take my finals, but then I want to go on and specialize in dermatology." He is looking through the rain into the distance. "I think it was those TV reports of the casualties in Vietnam – you know, the children with terrible burns from napalm bombs as well as the wounded American GIs. Some of them have horrifying injuries that have scarred them for life. A lot of research is being done in that field at the moment. That's something I'd like to get involved in." She sees that the grey in his eyes has deepened, becoming more intense. "It's weird. I don't know you but I'm telling you things I've never talked about with anyone before."

They sit in silence for a while, listening to the steady

rainfall. After his words, Holly is afraid of saying anything that may sound banal, but her curiosity overcomes her.

"Which university are you at?"

"London. I'm only here till the end of the week."

She would love to find out where he is staying and is working out a way to ask without appearing too inquisitive, when he speaks again.

"Do you know London?"

"No, I've never been." How can she explain that it is her dearest, wildest dream to study at the Slade School of Fine Art? But what did he just say about having a goal, not losing sight of your dream? "Perhaps I'll get there one day." She tries to sound more hopeful than she feels.

He is rising to his feet. The storm has ceased as suddenly as it began, the wind has died down and patches of clear blue fleck the sky. "We'd better see if we can get you away from here before the rain comes on again. Lean on my arm and try to put as much weight on me as you can."

Neither speaks as they slowly make their way over the moor to where the rugged hillside drops into the green dale below. Holly clings to his arm as they slip and slither downwards on the wet grass until they reach the bottom. Despite the pain in her foot she feels a deep sense of disappointment when they reach the gate to Black Ridge Farm, which he opens for her.

"I think your ankle will be alright if you rest it for a while, but maybe you should see a doctor – a qualified doctor, I mean – just to be sure." He hands her the easel. "Here's your equipment. I'm sorry about your painting, but don't give up."

"Thanks for everything. Won't you come in?"

He shakes his head. "I've got to be getting back. They'll be wondering where I've been." He smiles, turns abruptly and sets off, his dog racing ahead. Holly wonders for a moment who 'they' can be. He looks back and gives her a casual wave of his hand before he turns the bend in the lane and is gone from view.

Holly limps painfully towards the house, hoping her mother is out seeing a client. She needs some time to herself, time to go over her encounter on the moors, before she can share her experience with anyone.

"Well? What happened next?" Wide-eyed, Flo stares in anticipation. "Go on, Holly," she moans. "You can't leave me in suspense like this!"

Holly is gazing out of her bedroom window, her back towards her friend sitting on the bed. Her eyes stray over the hills that rise to the dark crags on the moors. Flo pounds the rose-patterned quilt savagely in her frustration.

"Really, Holly! You are the world's worst storyteller! Who on earth was your gorgeous knight errant? Where did this Nick come from? And where did he go? He can't just have vanished into thin air."

"I've no idea, Flo. Really I haven't. He just appeared from nowhere with this dog at his side. He must be staying somewhere round here, perhaps on one of the farms – but he didn't look as if . . ." Her voice trails off.

"You're hopeless!" Flo collapses among the roses on the bed in mock desperation. "Look, this conversation's getting us nowhere. It's time I brought you back to earth. Have you heard about Saturday? There's a great Rhythm 'n' Blues group from Leeds playing in Ainsley town hall. Shall we go? It would be fantastic to hear some live music for once."

"I know. Mike told me about it." Holly turns just in time to see the hurt on her friend's face. How could she have been such a fool as to mention Mike's invitation? Poor Flo! Mike is always nice to her, but he never looks at her the way he looks at Holly. Yet Flo is the dearest, most loyal person Holly can imagine. Why does he not realize that? Why does he not notice the beauty of her sweet face and womanly figure? She can see how Flo's calm and sunny disposition would fit the cheery outgoing temperament of a farmer's son. Unlike herself, Flo seems made for a life in the dales, a life determined by the steady passing of the seasons – ploughing, sowing, lambing, harvesting – and the never-ending farmhouse routine – washing-day, market-day, baking-day.

Holly crosses the little room to place a comforting arm round her friend's shoulders. "Let's all go on Saturday. If we go together, we'll have a great time."

She can guess what Flo's answer will be, but at that moment her mother calls from downstairs. "The dress is finished now, love. Just the hem to be turned up. I told Georgina it'd be ready by three so they're sending the car for you to take it over. It should be here any minute now."

Flo scrambles off the bed at once. "Is that the dress you designed for Georgina Ranleigh? Can I see it before you go?"

Holly smiles. "Well, 'designed' sounds a bit grand. She asked Mum to make her something special for a party because she couldn't find what she wanted in the shops. None of Mum's patterns seemed to match the material she had, so I did a sketch of what I thought would suit her and she liked it. That's all really. I cut it out but Mum has done all the sewing. She was up half the night getting it finished."

They go down into the sitting-room where the dress is hanging on a tailor's dummy. The cream, wild Thai silk shimmers in the lamplight. The tiny stitches at the seams and neckline are invisible to the naked eye, but it is the style that takes Flo's breath away. It is strikingly simple, but even on the dummy the intricate cut and cleverly hidden shaping combine to achieve a purity of line that is far from the fussy fashions of the day.

"It's gorgeous!" Flo stands open-mouthed. "I suppose they have dresses like that in London, but I've never seen anything like it round here, not even in York."

There is a sound outside and a sleek black Rover draws up in the farmyard. Holly meticulously wraps the dress in layers of tissue paper and holds it carefully as she goes out to put it on the back seat of the car. Jock, the chauffeur, was a friend of her father's and has known her since she was a child. Promising to phone Flo later, she gets into the front seat beside him and they set off for Ranleigh Hall.

"Jock," Holly begins tentatively as the car purrs down the

lane leading into the town, "how long have you been working for the Ranleighs?"

"Now let me see, lass." Jock pauses to shift the gears before going on in the soft burr of his Yorkshire accent. "My family's been in service at the Hall since my grandfather were a lad. I started work there in the greenhouses when I were fifteen. Of course they had plenty of servants then and when they needed a new chauffeur, I took on the job."

"And Lady Ranleigh? When did she have the accident? What happened?"

"Tragic it were. Fell off a horse she did. Nearly killed herself. It were just after Miss Georgina were born. 1942, I guess." Jock sighs at the recollection.

"When I was at the Hall last time, I had this feeling that there was something sad about the family. Do you think Lady Ranleigh and her husband were happy together?"

Jock gives her a quizzical look out of the corner of one eye. "What tales have you been listening to, lass? Far be it from me to say, but he had a roving eye did Gerald Ranleigh. Lady Marianne were a right beauty, and titled too. Deb of the year in one of the last London seasons before the war. Swept her off her feet he did. He were always quite a lady-killer. She came from a very wealthy family down south, proper landed gentry they were."

"The Ranleighs made their money fairly recently, didn't they?"

"That's right. Gerald's grandfather earned himself a huge fortune with iron works on the Tees at the end of the nineteenth century, but his only son, Gerald's father, were a gambler and frittered it all away before he died, leaving a load of debts, so I suppose Gerald had to marry money."

"Didn't he love Marianne?"

"I dare say he did, in his fashion. But it weren't long after the wedding before he had me driving him to certain establishments down Middlesbrough way, and after her accident he went out practically every night."

"What happened to him?"

"I suppose the good life took its toll because he liked his food and his drink as well. Died of a heart attack about eight years ago, he did."

"So Lady Marianne has been on her own ever since."

Jock shrugs his shoulders. "Eh, lass, she were on her own for a long while before then."

When the car pulls up in front of Ranleigh Hall it is Georgina herself who opens the door. She must have been watching for their arrival. Excitedly she leads Holly up the great sweep of the staircase to her bedroom, which is large and prettily decorated in shades of blue. The windows give onto a garden that stretches down to a lake surrounded by willow trees.

Georgina is already pulling off her skirt and sweater. She slips the dress over her head. "It's perfect." She smiles at her reflection as she turns slowly before the long mirror. "I couldn't have had it made up better in London, even if I'd been able to leave Mother to go. Please tell your mother, you've both done a wonderful job."

At Georgina's feet, Holly appraises her design, her brows drawn. The cut is just as she envisaged. The dress moulds itself faultlessly to Georgina's slim figure, creating an effect of softness despite the heaviness of the fabric. Her shining blonde hair exactly matches the sheen of the silk. Any addition, any change now would spoil it.

"I'll just fix the length," she mumbles through a mouthful of pins and begins to turn up the hem. She feels that this dress needs a hemline that is slightly higher than normal, just above the knee. Georgina turns patiently as she bends to her task.

"I wanted to ask you and your friends who sang for us the other night whether you'd like to come to my party on Saturday. It's my twenty-first and some people are coming down from London as well as a few girls I was at school with. Quite a crowd, but if you'd like to come, you'll all be very welcome. Then you'll be able to see me wearing your dress for the first time!"

Holly can barely gulp her acceptance. An invitation like this far outshines any concert in the town hall. She can hardly wait to tell the others. Her thoughts are racing as she wraps the dress in its tissue paper again to take it home for her mother to stitch the hem. A party, music and dancing . . . but what will she wear? Here heart sinks as she mentally reviews her wardrobe. She has nothing, absolutely nothing, that even remotely matches Georgina's dress. Her head is full of designs but she can only put them down on paper. Silk and chiffon, lace and velvet are not commodities to be found in a dales farmhouse.

When she gets into the car again, Jock notes her change of mood and stays silent. As they make their way back down the drive, a flash of red catches Holly's attention. A red MG is parked on the grass verge with its bonnet raised, its owner's head hidden as he delves into the engine. It looks just like the car whose reckless driver nearly rammed them the night they were out carol-singing. Holly turns in her seat, craning her neck to get a glimpse of him as they go past. Faded jeans over black leather boots jolt her into recognition. Nick! What is he doing here? Any doubt in her mind vanishes at the sight of a border collie that comes bounding across the lawn and leaps up joyfully to greet its master.

"Fine dog that," Jock nods admiringly. "Always fancied one myself but the missus wouldn't hold with it."

"Who does it belong to?" Holly's voice sounds strange in her ears.

"It's Nicolas Ranleigh's. Didn't you see him now, tinkering with that car of his? Eh lass, maybe you wouldn't recognize him. He's Georgina's brother. A couple of years older, I reckon. Not that us folks see a lot of him. Always at boarding school he were, and now he's studying to be a doctor in London. I expect he's here for the young miss's party on Saturday."

When his passenger does not reply, Jock turns his attention to the road. Darkness has fallen. Snowflakes swirl out of nowhere to splatter onto the windscreen. Holly finds her heart beating in time to the steady swish of the wipers. Thoughts are flying wildly through her head at the thought of seeing Nick again, but before long her common sense reins them in. In real life, princes do not have to rely on finding kitchen maids whose rags become ball gowns at the wave of a magic wand. There are already quite enough modern-day princesses who wear Mary Quant originals and drive their own Mini Coopers.

Yet a tingle of anticipation runs through her at the thought of the invitation and she cannot help wondering what the evening will bring.

Rovers and Jaguars far outnumber the Mini Coopers parked outside the Hall on Saturday evening. While Dave nudges his battered Morris between two gleaming limousines, Holly and her friends glance apprehensively towards the great house. On their last visit it was shrouded in darkness, but now light spilling from its tall windows makes it look even more imposing. The air is reverberating to the thudding rhythm of what, even at this distance, Dave announces to be a first-rate R&B group.

As they pass into the entrance hall, Georgina catches sight of them and leaves a chattering group of guests to greet them, both hands outstretched in welcome.

"It's great to see you! I'm so pleased you could all come. Annie will take your coats, then you can meet some of my friends." Graceful and relaxed, she flashes Holly an especially warm smile.

Holly hands her coat to the housekeeper almost reluctantly, conscious of the contrast between Georgina's gown and her own. She has done her best to alter the bridesmaid's dress she wore at a distant cousin's wedding the previous year, lowering the neckline, removing the sleeves and shortening it, but though the pale shade of peach matches her creamy skin and dark hair, the cheap satin is stiff and rustles when she moves. Her friends do not seem to be much at ease either, with Flo smoothing her long black skirt over her hips, Dave tugging at the knot of his tie and Mike intently studying his brown shoes.

Georgina leads them gaily through the guests thronging the hall into a large room where the carpets and furniture have been removed to create a dance floor. Huge boughs of holly, clusters of mistletoe and trailing ivy hang from the walls. Candles flicker on little tables round the gleaming parquet. At the far end, double doors have been thrown open to reveal a chef presiding over a magnificent buffet. At that moment the band strike a final chord on their guitars and stop for a break. Couples move to form groups, conversing loudly, joking and laughing. Their clothes, their accents, even their gestures match the cars outside; they seem so polished and self-confident. Flo, Mike and Dave move closer together. When a passing waiter offers them champagne, Holly takes a glass and finds herself clutching its fragile stem so tightly that she is afraid it may snap.

"Hi, Cathy! How's life on the moors these days?"

She almost spills her drink as she spins round to face him. Laughing grey eyes look down into her own. The floor sways beneath her feet, the clamour of voices recedes to a distant murmur and she feels a deep flush mount her cheeks. An eternity passes in which she knows she should say something – a clever riposte, an introduction to her friends, even a simple 'hello' would do, but the words will not come.

"Nick, have you and Holly met before?"

It is Georgina's voice that breaks the silence. Dimly Holly hears Nick's explanation followed by her friends' reactions, then his voice again asking her a question and, as if spoken by someone else, her own sounding amazingly calm and clear.

"Thanks, it healed very quickly. It was only a sprain."

The concern in his eyes vanishes, the smile returns and he seems about to speak. The group have started to play again, one of her favourite blues songs, and the slow pulsating rhythm makes her blood tingle with the longing to dance. Will he ask her? She hardly dares breathe for hoping.

"Shall we dance?"

It is Mike's voice. She bites back her disappointment. With a parting smile and a friendly nod in her direction Nick turns away. Her last glimpse is of his fair hair curling to touch the collar of his dinner jacket before he disappears into the crowd.

Holly bends her head to Mike's tweed-clad shoulder as they dance. She must enjoy this evening for its own sake and stop indulging in fantasies. During the slow love-song she can feel him pulling her closer. Flo has gone to the bar with Dave but Holly can sense her friend's unhappiness.

When the music stops at last, she suggests to Mike that they join the others. They reach them just in time to see Nick step onto the dance floor with one of the most stunning girls Holly has ever seen. Her swinging bob of auburn hair gleams like burnished copper and her white skin flushes with exertion as they rock to a pounding rhythm. Her red lips part to flash a brilliant smile at her partner whenever she turns towards him. The pale blue silk of her outrageously short dress whips softly round her slim hips over long legs that taper to elegant silver sandals. Tiny diamonds at her throat and ears catch the light and refract it a thousand times.

"Steady, old thing." Flo puts her arm round Holly's shoulders and gives her a sympathetic squeeze. "I've just been talking to Georgina. That's Nick's girlfriend, Caroline von Minter. Her father's a Harley Street consultant, a world-famous dermatologist in fact. Got the message?"

Holly takes a deep breath. "Got it. Come on, Flo. Have you seen that buffet? It's not often we country girls get to feast on smoked salmon and vol-au-vents. Let's forget that diet of yours. Just for tonight!"

They do not stay long. Soon after midnight Holly is home where she finds Elizabeth still bent over her sewing.

"Did you have a nice time, love?"

"Yes, Mum. It was . . . ," she pauses, looking for the right word, ". . . different."

In her room she stands at the window, looking out into the darkness. One day, she knows, her life will be different too. One day she will leave the dale. One day she will go somewhere really grand, and when she does she will be wearing a dress far lovelier than anything she has seen at Ranleigh Hall tonight.

FIVE

Paris, Spring 1967

The 'little something' which Arlette had in mind for Holly to wear at the opera was a sheath of white silk crêpe de Chine which bore a discreet tag with the name 'Saint-Laurent'. Falling softly from one shoulder while leaving the other bare, the dress moulded itself so perfectly to her figure that the seamstress who delivered it had scarcely any alternations to make.

As Holly stepped from the limousine in front of the Opéra, a slight evening breeze swirled the delicate fabric around her golden sandals, and the setting sun glinted on the gold and pearl clasp which Marie had placed in her upswept hair. The admiration in Julien's eyes as he came to greet her, elegant in a midnight-blue dinner jacket, added to Holly's confidence. Raising her head, she laid one hand lightly on his arm as he led her up the steps behind Arlette, who was resplendent in black lace over taffeta, with diamonds at her throat, and escorted by Comte Maurice de Villiers.

After they had taken their seats in their box, Arlette and Maurice nodded in acknowledgement to numerous acquaintances on all sides of the house, while Holly, seemingly intent on studying her programme, felt rather than saw the many curious glances directed at herself.

"Ma chère," Arlette whispered, bending towards her, "you are the sensation of the evening. All Paris is guessing at who you are!"

Holly felt a frisson of excitement run down her spine. She fell silent as the lights slowly dimmed and darkness enveloped them.

"If only they knew," she thought to herself, "they would not believe it." But then, she realized, she herself did not really believe what was happening either.

The overture began and she leaned forward in her seat, caught up in the beauty of the music. When the first act drew to a close she remained entranced, her surroundings forgotten.

"A glass of champagne, perhaps?" Julien's voice broke the spell. She turned hastily to face him, seeing that her companions had already risen to their feet for the intermission.

"Yes, thank you," she managed to reply, "that would be lovely."

Arlette and Maurice had joined friends in the next box where they were deep in a discussion on the merits of the singers. Julien led her to a foyer where waiters were serving drinks and canapés. Holly stood near an open window, enjoying the fresh air and hoping to escape the chatter and bustle of the other spectators so that the magic might linger a little longer. When Julien came over to her he was carrying two glasses of champagne. He gave one to her, then raised the other. His black eyes met hers.

"To you, Holly," he said softly, saying her name for the first time.

"Julien," she said simply, raising her glass to him. His eyes dwelt on hers for a moment longer, then on her lips as they touched the rim of her glass. She took a sip, allowing the delicious cool liquid to slip down her throat. Deep inside she felt a sudden stirring of feelings she had not experienced for more than two years.

The bell ringing to announce the end of the intermission punctuated her thoughts. As Julien led her back to their box amid the other spectators thronging to take their seats, her hand rested lightly on his sleeve. Was it the champagne, she wondered, that made her so acutely conscious of his muscular forearm under the fine fabric of his dinner jacket? When he pulled back her chair for her, his hand accidentally brushed her bare shoulder and she felt a thrill like an electric current run through her body.

During the second act she tried hard to concentrate on the action on the stage, but the haunting beauty of the music and the tragic story of the opera drew her thoughts elsewhere.

The rest of the evening flew by in a haze. It was a dream in which she knew she was dreaming and never wanted to awake. When, in the early hours of the morning, she at last lay in bed in her room, images flashed like snapshots into her mind. She saw the four of them crowding, laughing, into Arlette's limousine after the performance, then the luxurious dark-red interior of the famous restaurant and, inside, Maurice's joking refusal of the head waiter's suggestion of caviar and blinis and his insistence instead on pasta to complement their evening of Italian culture. The idea had been rapturously greeted by his companions and they had subsequently enjoyed a superb dish of buttery fettucine sprinkled with white truffles and parmesan. The impromptu supper had ended with a perfect zabaglione with yet more vintage champagne, and it had been long past midnight before the evening had drawn to a close.

Holly's last recollection before she drifted into sleep was how Julien had opened the door of the car for her, taken her hand to help her out and drawn her to him, kissing her lightly on both cheeks in the French manner while breathing the words "Tu es ravissante, you have enchanted me" so softly that she was uncertain whether she had really heard them.

It was nearly noon the next day when a timid knock at her bedroom door woke her from a deep sleep. It was Marie, but instead of the usual tray she was carrying an armful of flowers.

"Bonjour, mademoiselle. You wish for breakfast? These have arrived for you." She laid a magnificent sheath of white camellias on the bed.

Holly stared in amazement. She had never in her life received so much as a bunch of daffodils from anyone before. A calling card embossed in silver was tucked among the glossy green leaves. *Julien de Mervais* she read. There was no message.

The following Wednesday evening was one of the rare occasions when there were no guests for dinner. Holly and

Arlette were sitting in the drawing-room when the phone rang.

"Ma chère, it's for you."

Holly looked up in surprise. She seldom got any calls. Flo on her tight student budget always preferred to write letters and Holly did not have many contacts in Paris. She was so caught up in her work that she had little time or opportunity for making new friends and knew very few of the numerous British people living in the city. In fact she did everything to avoid them; any meeting would inevitably have led to comparing memories of England and she could not have borne being reminded of all she had lost.

She flushed slightly on hearing Julien's voice at the other end of the line. They had not spoken in the days that had passed since the night at the opera. Arlette had made no comment on the camellias he had sent her. Perhaps it was simply normal in these circles to send flowers after an evening out, Holly thought, but then she remembered those dancing black eyes and his parting words.

"Bonsoir, Julien." She tried to keep her voice light and steady. "Thank you so much for the lovely flowers."

"It is I who have to say thank you for such a wonderful evening." His voice was like black velvet. Arlette had discreetly withdrawn from the salon. She was tired after a long day at the office and signalled that she was going to bed.

"Bonne nuit, Madame," Holly called to her, one hand held over the receiver.

Meanwhile Julien was chatting in easy, almost familiar tones, quite different from the rather formal manner in which he had always spoken to her until now. "Will you come out with me tonight? There's a wonderful new club on the Left Bank, everybody's talking about it. I'd like to take you there."

"I'd love to, Julien," she replied, thinking quickly, "but not tonight. I'm exhausted. We had deadlines to meet at work today." She heard his ill-concealed sigh of disappointment. "Perhaps tomorrow evening?" she added.

His perfect manners gained the upper hand as ever. "Of

course. I understand. I'll pick you up at ten tomorrow. It's not far. In Saint Germain. We can easily walk there. Bonne nuit." There was a click at the other end. Without waiting for her reply he was gone.

Holly replaced the receiver thoughtfully. She was not particularly tired, but there was something about Julien which suggested that he was used to getting his own way where women were concerned. She loved the idea of going to the Rive Gauche for the evening, but in her time, not his.

Another reason, though Holly found it hard to admit, was that she felt she should tell Arlette first. How ridiculous, she thought. I'm twenty-two, I can do whatever I like. But she knew that was not the case in the Parisian high society to which Arlette belonged. The Swinging Sixties had not reached France. Holly had lived there long enough to see that girls from upper-class families did not go out alone after dark unless accompanied by a brother or trusted male friend. Flo's letters had told her of the effect that the contraceptive pill was having on students' behaviour at her college in York, but in Catholic France it was not available. Whispered comments had taught her that an unwanted pregnancy was a catastrophe, not just for the girl herself but also her family. Arlette had even mentioned that marriages in the upper echelons of French society were sometimes arranged at special parties known as 'rallies' where girls were introduced to suitable partners.

Holly did not for a moment expect Arlette to impose such strict standards of behaviour on her, but as a guest in her house she thought it best to tell her about Julien's invitation beforehand, even though she knew that Arlette would not oppose her accepting it. When she did so next morning, Arlette's response assured her that her intuition had been correct.

In the evening Julien appeared after dinner when the little ormolu clock in the salon was just chiming ten. Casual yet elegant in a white linen shirt, open at the neck, with a black cashmere sweater slung nonchalantly round his shoulders, he looked even more attractive than on the night of the opera. 'Devilishly handsome', Holly thought, recalling a phrase she had once read in a romantic novel. As he bent to kiss her lightly on both cheeks, she caught the masculine scent of his eau de toilette. When he complimented her on her appearance, she was glad she had finished making the soft grey flannel trouser suit, which she now wore with a silk shirt of the palest pink.

Julien put his arm around her to guide her as they made their way through the crowds thronging the Boulevard St Germain. The mild evening had drawn thousands of Parisians and tourists alike into the pavement cafés. The babble of their voices, the sounds of the traffic and the music of the street entertainers working their way past the outside tables mingled in their ears.

"Voilà!" Julien suddenly announced. Grasping Holly's arm he led her down a short flight of steps into a basement. The man on the door greeted Julien by name and stuffed the note he gave him into his back pocket. The cellar room was windowless, heavy with cigarette smoke and lit only by flickering candles. They were shown to a small side table with two chairs which must have been reserved since every other seat was taken.

As they sat down, the buzz of conversation ceased and clapping broke out as a tall slender woman in a long-sleeved black gown mounted a tiny dais. Somewhere a pianist struck a chord and she began to sing, not jazz as Holly had expected, but a chanson. Her deep melodious voice and the haunting dark eyes in her pale face were so expressive that she scarcely needed the gestures of her white hands that moved as if detached from her body. Les Feuilles Mortes; she sang of love dying like autumn leaves falling from the trees or footprints in sand being effaced by the wind. As the last notes faded away the audience sat still, caught up in her spell until a frenzied clapping broke out.

"It's Juliette Gréco, isn't it?" Holly's eyes shone in the candlelight. "I can't believe I'm here, seeing her in person. Thank you, Julien." In response Julien reached out and squeezed her hand. When the next chanson began, he left his hand covering hers.

On the evening that followed he took her to dine at La Tour d'Argent, one of the most exclusive and expensive restaurants in Paris. At his insistence she enjoyed some of the greatest dishes that French cuisine could offer, accompanied by the finest wines. Holly could not help asking herself why Julien should be lavishing so much attention and money on her. Educated at one of the 'Grandes Écoles', France's élite universities, and having travelled widely in the Far East, he had a wealth of knowledge and experience far superior to her own, but he seemed to like her company. At first she wondered whether he minded that they sometimes took the roles of teacher and pupil, but soon she saw that he enjoyed it. After long, tiring days in the office proof-reading articles for Arlette, she began to look forward to the stimulating times she and Julien spent together.

The next Saturday was reserved for the Louvre where Julien was most insistent that they should visit the ancient Egyptian and Greek collections before looking at the paintings. "Only tourists make a bee-line for the Mona Lisa." When they finally went to see Da Vinci's masterpiece, it was so small, almost insignificant beside the other great works of art, that Holly would have walked straight past had she not been alerted by the hive of Japanese swarming around it. She found a spot from where she could view the portrait of the world's most enigmatic woman. She looked so serene and content. What secret did that smile hold? No one would ever know. La Giaconda had taken it to her grave long ago.

Julien came to stand close behind her. "I think she has found the man she loves." His eyes were fixed on the painting but his words were for her. "But maybe she hasn't realized it yet," he added softly before moving away.

After leaving the Louvre they walked in silence, hand in hand, along the Tuileries until they reached the pond, where they sat down on a bench together. It was a bright, breezy afternoon and children were sailing boats on the sparkling water. The tiny wooden yachts were clearly for hire as they were exactly matching in size and shape, their coloured sails harmonizing in muted tones of blue, green and ochre. How Parisian, Holly thought. There was not a single plastic speedboat to be seen. No garish reds or yellows marred the scene. The miniature craft bobbed in the sunlight like an Impressionist painting. Under the watchful eyes of parents and nannies in the background, even the beautifully dressed little boys and girls seemed to be part of the picture.

Holly took a deep breath of the crisp clean air. "Julien, I don't know how to thank you," she began.

"Thank me?" he looked at her questioningly, almost as if he thought she might be joking. "What do you want to thank me for?"

"I know it sounds silly to say so, but I really feel I'm sort of completing my education here. I never really learned that much at school." She smiled ruefully at the recollection. "My head was always full of other things than what the teachers were trying to tell me. But the worst thing is, I even thought that what they were trying to tell me was all I needed to learn. I thought that if I knew enough maths and history and geography and so on, I'd be an educated person. But that's not true. It's only now that I'm starting to learn properly what life is all about. I was a child when I came here, but now I feel at last I've started to grow up. Thanks to you," she added shyly.

Her words seemed to touch him. He dwelt on them for some moments before he replied. "Please don't think that I felt you were uneducated. It's just that I want to show you all the things that mean so much to me. It doesn't matter whether it's music or art, food or wine, theatre or architecture – I just want to share all the things I know and love with you. My city, my culture," he added.

Holly realized that their conversation was taking a direction that she had not intended. She loved Paris and Parisian life but it was not her city. Perhaps it never would be, never could be. Her home had been in England, in a lonely dale where the wind swept down from the moors. Her time in Paris would be an important season of her life, but like all seasons it would come and go. She wondered if perhaps Julien wanted to say more than she was ready to hear?

She jumped to her feet, pretending to be cold, stamping her boots on the gravel and clapping her hands for warmth. Julien was instantly solicitous. She must not catch a chill on any account. He would take her at once to a salon de thé for some hot chocolate and on the way there he would tell her something about French theatre. Tucking her arm under his own, he led her down the long allée towards the Rue de Rivoli.

As they sat warming their hands around their bowls of steaming chocolate with a silver dish of rich dark truffles on the table between them, Julien talked about the famous Comédie Française and its origins in the Italian Commedia dell'Arte. Holly listened fascinated as he told her about the great playwright Molière. "I'll get tickets for us to see L'Avare tomorrow evening. You'll love it."

She wondered briefly why he had not asked her first whether she would like to see the play or not, but brushed the thought aside. After all, she had shown such interest, it was only natural that he should want to take her to the most famous theatre in Paris, and in any case she was really looking forward to the occasion.

She was not to be disappointed. After a magnificent performance at the Comédie Française they were crossing the little footbridge over the Seine on their way back to Arlette's apartment on the Ile Saint-Louis. Behind them Notre Dame rose into the darkness, silhouetted against the starlit sky, a huge galleon in the moonlight. Holly stopped to lean over the railing and look at the river below. She always loved to stand there in the evening, watching the lights of the bateaux-mouches with their cargoes of tourists slipping past, gliding over the smooth black water. Julien took her hand and they walked in silence till they reached the gates of the courtyard that led to Arlette's apartment.

"How lucky I am to be here, to have met Arlette, and you, and to be in this beautiful city." She raised her eyes to meet his but his face was in darkness. "It's like a fairy tale and I'm a princess. Je suis princesse." Her words sounded naïve but he did not laugh.

"Moi, roi, I am your king," he murmured. He stepped forward and took her in his arms. His mouth sought hers. She felt his tongue forcefully pushing her lips apart, his body pressing hard against her own. His arms seemed like iron bands encircling her. Suddenly she could not breathe. She could not bear his embrace. Summoning all her strength she pushed him away and he stepped backwards into the shadows. At that moment a light went on in the concierge's lodge. She said nothing but turned from him, slipped through the gates into the silent courtyard and ran up the stone steps to the doorway. When she looked back, he had already vanished into the night.

Without waiting for the lift, she raced up the ten flights of stairs to the apartment. Her thoughts were in turmoil. On reaching her room she flung herself onto the bed and lay there face down, her heart pounding with exertion and emotion. What was it that she wanted? If only she knew. Half of her body was crying out for Julien's caresses, wanting to feel the taste of his lips again. The recollection of the pressure of his body against hers made her feel weak. But there was something else there too, a barrier, an obstruction. Her heart could not respond to the call of her senses.

A vision which she had subdued and repressed for so long rose in her mind against her will. Grey eyes that crinkled when they smiled at her, tousled fair hair and a gentle English voice. She sat up slowly, her head in her hands. "No," she told herself fiercely. "No." She had tried so hard but even after all this time her feelings for him still stood between her and a relationship with another man. Julien was every girl's dream – charming and good-looking, cultured and intelligent, rich and, most important of all, seemingly bent on making her happy – yet the long fingers of the past were reaching out, grasping her, dragging her back, forcing her to remember what she could never forget . . .

SIX

North Yorkshire, Winter 1962-63

. . . December is one of the darkest periods of her life. During the short hours of daylight the skies periodically blacken to release yet another blinding snowstorm upon the moors. Vast sweeps of white level the landscape, covering hedgerows and fences, roads and signposts, a uniform blanket broken only by an occasional farmhouse roof. Deep drifts block the lane from Black Ridge Farm into the town.

Even when Tom Barton was alive, Christmas was a quiet time, and since his death Holly and her mother have spent it alone, simply enjoying each other's company and their reminiscences. Holly is never troubled by loneliness, and at the moment she has far greater worries. Elizabeth's cough has worsened and Holly hears her struggling to breathe at night, but her mother refuses to admit that she is ill. At Holly's insistence she has been to see Dr Westbury, returning home from his surgery with an assumed air of cheerfulness and as uncommunicative as ever when Holly tries to question her. The pills he prescribed do not seem to be helping her, but whenever Holly broaches the subject, Elizabeth always manages to divert her attention.

Holly's mind wanders anxiously as she rolls out pastry on the kitchen table for some mince pies. In the sitting room she can hear her mother opening boxes of Christmas ornaments so that she can decorate the tree which a kind neighbour brought them some days before. Perhaps she is worrying about nothing. She puts down the rolling pin and reaches for the pastry-cutter. When Spring comes, things are sure to get better . . .

A crash and a sharp cry rip though her thoughts. One moment she is frozen, immobile with fright, the next she is racing into the adjoining room. The tree is hanging oddly, diagonally in the air, its branches caught in the heavy curtains. The stepladder is splayed across the carpet, half hiding Elizabeth's inert form.

"Mum!" Holly hears her own voice shaking with fright. "Mum, are you alright?" Her palms still white with flour, she flings the ladder to one side and drops to her knees. She lifts her mother's head and pats her cheek but Elizabeth's eyes remain closed, her face deathly pale, her breathing shallow, barely discernible.

Holly scrambles to her feet and rushes to the phone. She must have dialled Flo's number a thousand times but never with such a wildly beating heart and such trembling hands.

"Mrs Westbury? It's Mum – she's had an accident. Please can Dr Westbury come over here at once . . ."

"I'm sorry, my dear. That's quite impossible."

Horrified, Holly forces herself to listen to the patient motherly voice at the other end of the line. The dale is cut off, the roads are impassable, the phone line to the hospital is down, the doctor out on an urgent case – a burst appendix – a matter of life and death. There is only one person whom she can think of who may be able to help, Mrs Westbury continues, the only one with any medical experience in the dale – Nicholas Ranleigh. He is home from medical school for Christmas. She will ring the Hall and ask him to go over, the calm resolute voice continues, soothingly. She gives Holly some brief instructions for first aid before hanging up.

Holly puts the phone down in dismay. Her mother needs expert medical attention, not a student whose main interests are fast cars and rich girls! Hearing a low moan from the sitting room, she rushes back and sees that Elizabeth has recovered consciousness. Her eyes are open and she is trying to get up. Holly half supports, half carries her mother up the steep staircase to her bedroom. By the time the doorbell rings, Elizabeth is lying under the covers, pale and protesting weakly at all the fuss on her account. Holly opens the front door almost unwillingly. She would rather wait for Dr Westbury than put herself in Nick

Ranleigh's debt once again. He should return to the London society where he belongs.

Was she really expecting a teasing smile and a joking remark? When Nick comes in, pulling off his anorak in a flurry of snowflakes, his manner is entirely professional. He enquires briefly about the accident and, before she has finished replying, is on his way up the narrow staircase, taking two steps at a time. Holly stands back as he examines her mother, gently bending each limb, carefully looking into her eyes and tapping her back and chest while he listens intently through his stethoscope. After he has examined a bottle of pills on the bedside table, he sits down on the bed and takes Elizabeth's hand in his while he asks her some simple questions.

Holly watches in bewilderment. Is this a man who is planning to marry his way into Harley Street? Perhaps she has been wrong. She sees how snow is still clinging to his jeans. He must have waded waist-deep through the drifts to reach them. Snowflakes in the curls at the nape of his neck are melting into droplets of water that glint in the lamplight before they drip unheeded into the collar of his flannel shirt. She remembers how gently he held her foot when she hurt her ankle on the moors, how earnestly he spoke of his vocation to use his medical skills. Somehow it does not all fit together. She no longer knows what to think. She turns away, leaving doctor and patient together. Downstairs in the kitchen she vigorously stokes the fire and puts a kettle of water on the range to boil. Better give him something hot to drink after he has come all this way in such weather. That is something even a hill-farmer's daughter can offer.

His footsteps sound on the stairs and he bends his head under the low jamb of the door as he enters. Not trusting herself to speak, Holly gestures towards one of the armchairs in front of the hearth. He sits down, his hands closing round a mug of hot coffee, and he takes a long drink before raising his eyes to hers. "You were right to call for help. She'll be pretty bruised and sore but she doesn't seem to have fractured anything. She should never have been on that step-ladder –"

"I know. But she's pretty determined sometimes." Holly smiles ruefully. For the first time since the accident she can feel the tension starting to ebb from her body.

"Sounds like someone else I know." Nick grins at her before his serious expression returns. "But she'll have to be more careful. Attacks of giddiness or even fainting are a common side-effect of those pills she's taking. She's very weak. In fact it'll be quite a while before she'll be able to get up at all. I'm sure Dr Westbury would like to have her in hospital for a check-up as soon as the roads are passable. How long has she been suffering from it?"

"The giddiness?" Holly looks at him questioningly. "It's new. She's never fainted before."

"No, I mean the tuberculosis itself." He goes back to drinking his coffee before he realizes that Holly's back is turned towards him, her shoulders shaking with emotion. In an instant he is on his feet, his arms around her. She buries her face in the soft wool of his sweater as wave after wave of shock and misery sweep over her. He holds her tightly till the huge sobs which rack her body have subsided. Eventually she raises her face to his to find that his eyes, searching her own, are filled with sympathy and regret.

"I'm sorry. How could I be so stupid? I thought you knew. I should never have . . ."

"No. I'm glad you told me," she whispers. "Somehow I've suspected all along that it was serious but I didn't want to admit it. It's better for me to know." Tears well up in her eyes again.

Gently he leads her back to the fireside and makes her sit down. He pulls his chair over to be close to her and, still holding both her hands tightly, one by one answers all her questions.

"She'll need a nurse. You can't possibly look after her and work as well. I'll see what Dr Westbury can arrange. And please, try not to worry. Those drugs are the best ones on the market. And the body itself has terrific powers to fight off illness."

His presence fills the room as they talk. While he is there she feels calmer. He gives her the strength she needs. But when he has left, swallowed up into a black void of swirling snowflakes, she realizes that she will probably never see him again.

She will have to face the future alone.

Winter continues to hold the dale in its icy grip during the first months of 1963. Early lambs born under the snow to moorland ewes die before they can be found. People cling to the warmth of their hearths, their lonely farmhouses huddling on the hillsides for shelter as storm after storm sweeps in off the North Sea to buffet the bare landscape.

Holly spends as much time at home as she can, but despite almost daily visits by Dr Westbury, Elizabeth seems unable to recover her strength. Frail but nonetheless stubborn, she refuses to go into hospital. Although exhausted by the routine of looking after her, Holly is unwilling to allow a stranger into the house to help. In the end it is at Dr Westbury's insistence, coupled with her own fear of falling ill, that she accepts a nurse, and Sally March arrives. It would be hard to find two persons less alike, the quietly-spoken, dark-haired farmer's wife and the bustling little nurse, her blonde curls turning grey, who, with an inexhaustible supply of energy and good humour, takes over their small household.

Sally has inherited what she calls 'a tidy fortune' from a maiden aunt and has given up her post at the hospital to be free, as she puts it, "to help where help is needed" in the local community. Holly is deeply grateful; she could never have afforded any nursing care for her mother. Now that Elizabeth can no longer take in sewing, money is very tight. Her wages and Elizabeth's tiny widow's pension have to support them both. Her secret hope of studying is out of the question. Her future seems as bleak as the landscape outside.

She glances over at the figure lying in bed, so thin that the blankets barely rise. Elizabeth's shallow but regular breathing means that she has slipped into a drugged sleep after a night that was long and painful. Her cough has become even worse despite a course of infusions which Dr Westbury thought might bring a change for the better. Turning her attention to the book in her lap, Holly suddenly hears voices in the kitchen below. She tiptoes past the bed, softly closing the door behind her, and goes down the narrow stairs, hoping the doctor has not chosen this time for his daily visit. She could not bear to wake her mother just now.

When she hears his voice, a thrill goes through her body. She pauses and struggles to appear composed before entering the room. She has not seen Nick since his last visit at Christmas when he held her in his arms to comfort her, an act which meant nothing, absolutely nothing at all. He must have returned to London soon after.

He is sitting beside the kitchen fire, balancing a mug of tea on one knee and chatting to Sally. He jumps to his feet on seeing her and she smiles back at him shyly.

"Hello. I just wanted to look in and see how your mother is, but I hear she's asleep."

"Yes, at last. I'm afraid she's really not too good at the moment."

They stand staring at one another in silence, neither knowing what to say until Sally comes over, takes each by the arm and gently propels them towards the back door. "Look here, Nick Ranleigh, you can't see Elizabeth but there's one good turn you can do while you're here and that's take this young woman out for a breath of fresh air. The roads are clear for the first time in weeks and I see you've got that car of yours outside. This lass does now't else but worry. That's a recipe for ill health if ever there was one, and I can't be doing with two invalids on my hands."

Nick smiles at Holly's unsuccessful protests as Sally thrusts her coat into her arms and firmly pushes them both over the threshold. "It doesn't look like we've got much choice, does it? Let's go then! How long is it since you've seen the sea?"

"Ages, I can't even remember when." She pulls on her coat. "I love the sea in winter."

"So do I." He opens the car door for her. "There's something wild and wonderful about it then."

Neither speaks as the car roars up the winding road leading out of the dale and speeds along the moorland ridge that runs towards the coast. Suddenly the broad sweep of the bay at Sands End comes into view. Holly gasps with delight. The pale blue of the winter sky blends so perfectly with the delicate grey-green of the sea that the horizon is no more than an indefinite line where the elements mingle. Black specks of fishing boats crawl like tiny insects along it, heading for the harbour of the ancient town of Whitby. Red-roofed cottages are scattered clumsily along both sides of a road that plunges precariously downhill until it reaches the little village on the shore, tucked into a crevice in the cliffs like a smugglers' hideaway.

At the bottom Nick turns the car into the empty car park and they sit gazing at the deserted beach. The holiday homes facing the sea are shuttered and abandoned, the kiosks boarded up for the winter. A faded poster for a long-past entertainment on the pier at Scarborough flutters forlornly in the wind. The tide is halfway out and a wet expanse of sand glitters before them in the cold winter sun. Holly jumps out of the car and the breeze tears at her dark hair as she inhales the salty air.

"Isn't it great? I'd forgotten what it's like to be here in winter. Can you smell the sea? It's so fresh and clean!"

She runs down the beach to the water's edge, leaving a trail of footprints that glisten in the wet sand. Caught by her enthusiasm, Nick follows her. He bends down and chooses several disc-like stones that have been ground smooth and flat by the force of the sea. Taking careful aim he sends them, one after another, skimming over the water, touching the surface once, twice, three, four times before they disappear beneath the waves. Holly laughs with delight and tries to copy him but fails at every attempt. Her pebbles refuse to bounce even once and simply vanish underwater with a resounding plop.

"Here. Let me show you." Standing behind her, he takes her right hand in his. Drawing her arm back together with his own, he then brings it forward to release a stone that flies smoothly, dipping to touch the surface of the water several times.

"Four jumps!" She cries out like a joyful child and swings round to face him in her excitement, but his hand is still holding hers. Suddenly she is in his arms and his eyes, grey like the sea, are above her. She hardly has time to draw breath before his lips descend, seeking her own, very gently at first as if to taste the salt of the sea air, then more insistently. The pounding of the waves on the beach, the crashing of the breakers out at sea and the screaming of the gulls overhead blend into a roar that fades when he whispers her name. She rests her head against his shoulder, burying her face in the warm folds of the scarf round his neck. Despite the thrill of their kiss she is perfectly calm. For the first time in weeks, cares no longer fill her thoughts. She is completely at peace.

Hand in hand they walk along the beach. It is as if they have always known each other. She finds herself telling him about her life at home, the farm, her mother, her dead-end job and her love of art. Nick listens intently and says little, but the expression in his eyes shows that he understands her fears and worries.

When she asks him about his own life, he speaks of his unhappy relationship with a choleric father he barely knew, his anger on realizing how his father's unfaithfulness was hurting his mother, how even as a little boy he wanted to protect her and help her. Through his words Holly sees that, despite his family's wealth and the grandeur of his home, he has never known the warmth and love that childhood should bring.

The tide is far out now. Several hours must have passed and the sea has turned a deep grey, reflecting ominous clouds that hang heavy overhead. The blustery wind has changed direction and is sweeping down from the north. "Time to go!" Nick announces, and they laugh, remembering the painting which brought them together. As they run for the car, thick snowflakes are starting to tumble from a rapidly darkening sky.

Inside, Nick leans over and gently brushes the snow from

Holly's hair before reaching for the ignition key. The engine splutters into life. The windscreen wipers swish a wet blanket of white aside. The headlamps cut through the gloom in search of the road that will take them back up onto the moors. At intervals the tyres rotate helplessly on the freezing surface as they begin the upward climb. Nick drives slowly, keeping up a steady pace. The bay falls away behind them in the gathering darkness. Lythe Bank lies before them, the steepest hill on the coastline, and they both know that once they have climbed it the journey home will be manageable.

At the bottom of the bank Nick engages first gear. Their visibility has been reduced to a few yards by what is now a driving blizzard. Gradually the car creeps forward. Inch by inch and foot by foot they crawl up the steep incline. Then suddenly red lights gleam faintly and a huge black shape looms ahead. Nick brakes and they slip backwards before slithering to a halt. In front of them an articulated lorry has failed in its attempt to climb the bank and is jack-knifed in their path, blocking the entire road.

Nick scrambles out of the car and is at once swallowed by the snowstorm. Holly joins him at the roadside where he is surveying the scene. There is no way they can pass.

"We'll have to turn round, go further down the coast and take a different route home." He curses mildly and takes her hand, but before they reach his car crunching tyres announce the arrival of a large removal van. Finding his route barred, the driver quickly slams on the brakes, causing the van to slew drunkenly until it comes to a standstill completely across the road. The driver revs the engine in repeated attempts to turn the van round but its tyres only spin helplessly on the icy surface.

"Oh no! It's blocked us in. We'll never get out of here now." Nick runs a hand in despair through his wet hair. A closer inspection confirms his fears: the MG is trapped between the two snow-bound vehicles.

"What are we going to do? I'm frozen already." Holly pulls her coat round her tightly in the biting wind. The cold of the icy road is creeping through the soles of her boots. The two other drivers are now in vehement dispute.

Nick shivers and turns up the collar of his coat. "If they ever stop quarrelling about whose fault it is, they're going to need a breakdown service to get them out of here. That could take hours. We'll freeze if we wait here that long."

"What are we going to do?"

"I've got an idea where we could shelter."

"Anywhere as long as we can get out of this snowstorm," Holly says, with more enthusiasm than she is feeling.

Still holding her hand, Nick leads her back down the icy slope. She slithers, slips, almost falls at times, but he steadies her until they reach the bottom. There they leave the road and turn into a narrow lane bordered by dense woods. Leafless trees stretch thick branches skywards, arching to form a cathedral of darkness and hiding a watery moon that has lighted their way till now.

"Where are we going?" Holly wonders aloud. There is no village in sight, no lamps beckon through the trees and no sound breaks the deep silence other than the rustle of the wind in the treetops and the distant hoot of an owl in hunt of prey.

"Don't look so frightened. We're just about there now. Only a few more yards from here, down by the stream." He is guiding her along an overgrown path, bending back tangled branches with snapping twigs that bar their way. The moon suddenly emerges from behind the clouds to reveal a small cottage. It must be two or three hundred years old at least, perhaps built for a farm worker and his family. Somewhere nearby she can hear the running water of a fast-flowing stream.

Nick is on his knees inside the porch. "This is our fishing cottage – my family's, I mean. We've had it for generations. We used to come here often when we were little. My father went trout-fishing. My sister and I used to play in the woods." He seems to be lifting up various flower pots and feeling inside them. "Here it is." He stands up, triumphantly holding an iron key. "Let's see if we can get in with this."

With a welcome click the latch snaps back. Nick flings the

door open. Since the inside of the cottage is as cold and dark as outside, Holly wonders whether she should feel relieved or not. Nick disappears into the blackness, overturning a chair on the way. She hears him strike a match. Within moments the soft yellow glow of a paraffin lamp fills the small room. He turns to face her and, although his face is in the shadows, she can tell from his voice that he is smiling. "It's not a palace, but at least it's a shelter."

He takes her hand and draws her inside . . .

SEVEN

. . . Holly steps over the threshold. After so little light outside it takes only a moment for her eyes to accustom themselves to the darkness inside. The door leads directly into a room where there is space for no more than a plain wooden table, two bentwood chairs, a worn sofa covered with red-patterned chintz, and a colourful rag rug in front of a tiled hearth. A fire of sticks has been set in the grate. Nick is already kneeling before it. He applies a match to the kindling and soon a trembling flame is licking the tinder until it crackles into life. He throws some logs onto the blaze and the strong scent of wood smoke pervades the room. In the flickering firelight Holly can also make out a staircase against one wall that perhaps leads to an upstairs bedroom. To the other side of the fireplace there is a door, possibly to a scullery at the back. The room smells musty and is as icy as the night outside; the cottage must have been empty for several years.

Suddenly she feels exhausted. The cold seems to have penetrated her whole body. She lets herself fall onto the sofa. It is surprisingly soft and comfortable. She pulls off her boots and stretches her feet out towards the fire hoping that its flames will begin to thaw her frozen limbs, but although it is already spreading a trembling half-circle of light, it has not even started to lessen the chill of the room.

"My feet are so numb I don't think I'll ever be able to walk again."

Nick turns from the fire to face her. The lamplight softens his features. He takes her feet in his hands and begins to massage them with slow, rhythmic pressure. She feels the blood flowing into her toes, which tingle to his touch. The memory of their first meeting on the moors comes flooding back, overwhelming her. A warm glow is spreading through her whole body.

"Come here," he whispers, gently pulling her downwards until she is beside him on the rug. Her back is against the sofa, the heat of the fire on her face. He draws her closer, and when he kisses her she sees his eyelashes descend to stroke his cheek. His lips touch her own, softly as he kissed her on the beach, but then more insistently. His hand is nestling in the hair at the nape of her neck, pulling her to him until his tongue is probing her slightly parted lips. She stiffens for a moment in hesitation. "Don't be frightened," he whispers softly. "I won't do anything you don't want me to do. You know I couldn't."

She feels his kisses on her cheek, her lips, her neck, her throat, tiny caresses yet each one thrilling her to the core of her very being. His fingers find the top button of her shirt and open it and she draws back slightly.

"Please, let me."

She nods imperceptibly, allowing him to slip her shirt off her shoulders and she feels the warmth and tenderness of his hand cupping her breast. Slowly he bends his head, his lips finding their way along her neck, across her throat and downwards to her nipple. His tongue begins to caress it deliciously, at first pulling gently, then almost biting as it hardens to him. She moans softly. The sound seems to excite him further, to heighten his desire to increase her pleasure. Her senses thrill to his touch. When she strokes the loose fair curls falling into his collar he raises his eyes to hers and – almost casually – whispers the words which she knows now she has been longing to hear. "You know, I think I'm falling in love with you."

"I think I know the feeling," Holly breathes. Her fingers reach for the buttons on his shirt and she opens them slowly, one by one, pressing her lips to his body as he draws her down towards him till they are lying entwined on the rug in the firelight.

Hours pass. Kisses and caresses, spoken and unspoken promises hold them together until she becomes drowsy and he is content to lie with her dark hair spilling over his shoulder, her body moulded perfectly to his own, to observe the darkness of her lashes against her pale cheeks and the soft rise and fall of her white breasts as she sleeps. He rises silently, taking care not to disturb her, and slips upstairs, returning with a large quilt with which he covers them both. As he does so, she moves towards him in her sleep and softly murmurs words he does not understand.

When he awakes, the fire has long gone out and a ray of watery light is filtering through the thin curtains. A chill dampness fills the room. The quilt has slipped and he reaches to pull it over them again, but this time the movement wakes her. She opens her eyes and smiles dreamily. "Nick Ranleigh, do you know what?"

"What? Tell me." He kisses the top of her head and looks down at her.

"I'm starving, and dying of thirst as well!"

He laughs and gets to his feet. "Then I'd better see what I can find here." Shivering with cold, he pulls on his clothes and disappears into the scullery at the back of the cottage.

"Mm . . ." Enjoying the warmth of the place where his body has been, Holly snuggles down under the quilt. "I'll have some nice hot coffee, please, and toast with honey – oh yes, and a glass of fresh orange juice as well."

"Certainly, miss, I'll see what I can do."

She hears him moving around, striking a match to light a stove and then the clatter of a saucepan. Some minutes later he returns with two mugs and holds one out to her. "Sorry, but I'm afraid this is the best I have to offer you!"

Holly takes it and sniffs the steaming red liquid inside. "Hmm. This is the first time in my life I've had tomato soup for breakfast." She looks at him mischievously over the rim as she sips. "But I can really recommend it."

"Well, it was either this or sardines. No tea or coffee, I'm afraid. The water pipes are completely frozen up. It's still just as cold as it was last night."

No sooner has he spoken than the words wrench Holly out of the dream she has been living in for the past hours. The spell they have woven together is broken. She is back in the real world and its worries flood into her mind, submerging her with such force that her fears tumble from her lips.

"What about the car? How soon can we get back? My mother will be frantic. She has no idea where I am. Can I at least phone her from somewhere?" She is on her feet, searching wildly for the clothes which they had cast aside only hours before.

Nick's first reaction is to comfort her. "Don't worry. I'm sure she'll have guessed what's happened. The snowstorm last night was the worst one so far this winter. We can't have been the only ones that didn't get home over the moors yesterday."

"Yes, but she'll be thinking we've had some terrible accident or something. She does worry so – you see, I'm all she's got." Her thoughts are completely centred on getting home now; he sees that they must leave at once.

Minutes later they are outside in the crisp morning air, in a world so beautiful that they can only gasp with wonder. Heavy white hoar-frost coats every branch, twig and blade of grass, sparkling in the sun that is shining from a sky of unbroken blue ice. Their breath hangs suspended in hazy clouds before their faces. Yet Holly's fears cast a long dark shadow over the winter magic of the scene.

When they reach the car, the other vehicles have gone, tyre-marks and footprints in the snow the sole trace of the events of the night before. Nick revs the engine and, after a moment of anxious waiting, it bursts into life.

The drive home seems to take longer than the journey of the previous day. The hours they have spent together now lie between, binding them together, yet at the same time forcing them to accept a changed situation which neither can entirely visualize.

Holly has fallen silent. Her eyes are swimming with tears that blur her vision of the road ahead. She dare not look at Nick lest he see them. The nearer they come to her home, the sooner the time they have spent together is drawing to an end. What role can she possibly play in his life – or he in hers? He must return to London, to university life with all its attractions. And she? She swallows hard at the thought of the job she must go back to on Monday morning. She surreptitiously wipes her eyes but Nick does not notice. His gaze is fixed on the road that runs along the bleak high ridge of moorland where drifts of snow alternate with patches of black ice. As the wind whistles past outside, he is speaking joyfully, insistently, of when he will see her again, making plans. She must come up to London to visit him and meet his friends. She can stay with him in his flat, his flatmate will not mind. They will go to some of the clubs he has been telling her about. There is a ball in the summer term, she must come up for that as well, she will love it. Of course, he will try to come to Yorkshire as often as he can at week-ends . . .

The treacherous condition of the road takes too much of his attention for him to be aware that she does not respond. They are nearing her home now. Familiar farms, cottages and fields stream past. Finally he pulls up at the gate of Black Ridge Farm and switches the engine off. He pulls her towards him and kisses her gently. "I'd better be off before the neighbours start gossiping."

"There are usually about thirty neighbours grazing in the meadow over there, but since they are all safely shut away in the barn at this time of year, you're saved from having to answer any embarrassing questions." Holly raises her hand and strokes his cheek.

"I'll call tomorrow to see you – and your mum, too. Take care." He lays a finger softly on her lips. No sooner has she slammed the car door behind her than he throws the engine into reverse gear, turns smartly in the narrow yard and vanishes round the bend in the lane with a roar.

Turning to the house, Holly lifts the heavy five-barred gate with both arms until it swings back on rusty hinges. What is she going to say to her mother? Somehow the question has never presented itself until now. How could she stay away all night without saying where she was? Elizabeth will have imagined that something terrible has happened. Holly hopes that Sally was able to calm her down. She is certainly going to have a lot of explaining to do and some awkward questions to answer, but her mother will understand, she is sure. Facing Sally will probably be worse. She has experienced the little nurse's sharp tongue and plain speaking on more than one occasion already.

"Mum, it's me. I'm back!" Her voice rings out as she lifts the latch on the back door and it creaks open. Even before she looks round the kitchen she senses that something is wrong. It is only secondarily that she feels the coldness in the little room. There is no one there. The kitchen fire which they bank up at night and always keep burning has gone out, the grate bare except for a few charred splinters of wood. Where has Sally gone? How could she possibly leave her mother alone like this?

"Mum! Are you alright? It's me!" She races up the narrow stairs taking them two at a time and flings open her mother's bedroom door. The room is in darkness and bitterly cold, the bed empty, its covers thrown back, the curtains still drawn. Spinning on her heel, she almost falls down the steep staircase in her haste to get back to the kitchen. A note, a message, there must be something! They cannot just have gone and left her alone like this! Yet already, even in her distress, a small voice inside her brain is telling her that it is she who left them, not the other way around.

Downstairs she sweeps one hand along the top of the high mantelpiece over the kitchen range, almost knocking off the clock and the pair of china candlesticks that her mother treasures. Nothing! She checks the dresser. No note is tucked between the rows of upright plates and dangling cups. Turning in panic she glimpses something white propped up against the teapot on the kitchen table. Like a fool she has overlooked the most obvious place. She snatches up the scrap of paper. It is clearly written in Sally's neat round hand but the words tumble over one another before her eyes. She sits down and forces herself to read them slowly.

Elizabeth had a sudden haemorrhage. Sally rang Dr Westbury who came and called an ambulance that took her to St.

Christopher's Hospital. But when? Holly stares at the note, turning it over. There is no indication of when it was written.

She tries to think calmly. She looks round for anything Elizabeth might need that Sally has forgotten. Her wash-bag is gone, as well as a small suitcase. On the bedside table she finds her mother's reading-glasses, and hanging on a hook on the back of the bedroom door, her worn blue dressing-gown. Holly holds it to her face for a moment before pushing it into a carrier bag with a few nightdresses. They must have left in a hurry for Sally, always so efficient, to have forgotten that.

Through the window she can see that it is beginning to snow again. She cannot afford a taxi. It never occurs to her to ring Nick and ask him to drive her into town. Instead she drags her bicycle out of the stables and starts the slippery descent down the icy lane towards the town and the hospital.

As she runs up the steps that lead to the entrance, she tries to suppress the thought that it is here that her father died. She is directed to a side ward where her mother is in a single room. She prays that this is the result of Dr Westbury's kindness and not necessitated by the severity of her mother's illness, but when she enters, she feels less hopeful.

Elizabeth is surrounded by equipment monitoring her vital functions. A tall metal cylinder supplying her with oxygen stands like a sentry beside the bed. A nurse adjusting a drip puts a warning finger to her lips when she sees Holly come in. "Only a minute," she mouths rather than says, "and don't say anything that might upset her." She picks up a tray of instruments and throws a practised glance round the room before leaving.

Holly approaches the bed. Her mother looks so slight, more fragile than ever. The whiteness of the sheets accentuates her pallor. Her skin seems transparent, almost bloodless, beneath the dark hair streaked with grey. Her breathing is so shallow that the bedclothes barely move.

"Mum, it's me, Holly." At her words Elizabeth's eyes open slowly and she smiles faintly but does not attempt to speak. With an effort she raises one hand an inch or two from the covers and

Holly takes it in her own, shocked by its coldness. As she gently rubs her mother's thin fingers, bare except for her worn gold wedding ring, she tries not to show her fear. "You'll be feeling better soon, Mum. The doctors and nurses will help you get well and strong again."

All at once Elizabeth becomes agitated. She lifts her head from the pillow and her breath comes in short gasps. In desperation Holly looks round for a bell to ring for the nurse, but cannot see one. She wants to go and get help, but her mother's grasp has tightened on her hand with an astonishing burst of strength.

"What is it, Mum? Just keep calm. Breathe slowly and you'll be alright," she says with more conviction than she is feeling. "Shall I call the nurse?"

"No." The single word is barely audible. Her hand is pulling Holly down until she is bending forward, her ear almost to her mother's lips. When Elizabeth speaks again, the words are less than a whisper. "There's something you have to know – now – before it's too late. No . . ." She resists Holly's attempt to restrain her from speaking further. "You know we loved you, Dad and I. We loved you more than anything else in the world. But . . ."

A fit of coughing overcomes her. Holly helps her take a sip of water. "Mum, please. Don't try to talk now. There's no need to . . ." But Elizabeth lifts a hand feebly to silence her and her eyes plead with her to listen.

"I should have told you long ago . . . somehow the time never seemed right. There is something you have to know. Before it's too late," she repeats, her breath coming in painful gasps. "You are not Tom's child. Your father was someone else. Tom knew, but he loved you as if you were his own child. Believe me, please. You were the little girl he always wanted." The dark-green eyes are begging her.

Holly bends as close as she can. "Oh Mum, of course I believe you. It doesn't make any difference. He'll always be Dad to me. I have never loved anyone like I've loved you and Dad." Elizabeth's eyes are going out of focus, clouding over. The fingers gripping her hand are losing strength. Holly's reason warns her against taxing her mother any further but although she summons all her will power, the words still tumble out. "Mum, tell me. I've got to know. If Dad was not my real father, who was?"

Seconds pass. Elizabeth is slipping from her. The hand which grasped Holly's own so urgently now gradually goes limp. The lids descend slowly over her dark-ringed eyes and only one word escapes her pale lips. "Philippe!"

Did Elizabeth answer her question or was she calling his name? Holly will never know. Only the bleeping of a monitor breaks the death-like silence in the room. She stares in horror at its screen, transfixed, then rushes into the corridor, calling for the nurse, who comes running. An angry look is thrown in Holly's direction before she is ordered out of the room. Around the bed there is a flurry of activity. She finds herself standing alone in the corridor, shaking.

The next hours drag by in a small waiting-room stuffed with wheelchairs, dismal furniture and tattered magazines. Sometimes she can ask one of the doctors or a passing nurse for news. On two occasions she is allowed to see her mother again, but Elizabeth's eyes remain closed and she does not react when Holly takes her hand.

Holly longs to ring Nick but something stops her. The joy of discovering his love for her and the memories of the night they have spent together have faded. Was it her fault that her mother suffered this attack? Was it brought on by the worry caused by her failure to return home? Is she to blame?

A young doctor comes in and sits down beside her. He offers her coffee in a paper cup. She takes it gratefully, realizing that she has not had anything to eat or drink since her unconventional breakfast with Nick.

"It's your mother in Room 12, isn't it?" he asks sympathetically.

She nods, unable to find the words to reply.

"Is there anyone you'd like to contact?"

Holly shakes her head. There is no one. She has no brothers

or sisters. Elizabeth's husband is dead, her parents, too, and her only relative, a cousin, lives in Scotland. Although she is well-liked in the town, she has no special friends. What a lonely life she has led. And yet she has always seemed content. "All she ever wanted was my happiness," Holly thinks, "and I let her down. When she really needed me, I wasn't there." Guilt creeps over her like black lava.

When she raises her head the doctor has gone, leaving her alone with her thoughts. "Please, God," she begs, "please let her live." When she was younger she went to church on various occasions and sat through countless assemblies at school, but until now religion has never had any particular meaning for her. "Please, God," she prays, "let her live and I promise . . ."

Her thoughts end there. What does she promise? What promise is big enough to warrant such a reward? And if God exists, surely He is not there to be bargained with? She gives up the attempt. All she can do is wait.

In the late afternoon Flo and Mrs Westbury arrive and gently persuade her to spend the night at their home. "Please, Holly," Flo pleads, "there's no more you can do here. You're just exhausting yourself."

"Come along, my dear," Mrs Westbury's no-nonsense voice cuts off further discussion. "We'll bring you back first thing in the morning. A good night's sleep is what you need now. The hospital will call us if there's any change."

Holly allows herself to be led away. She has lost the ability to make any decisions. At the Westburys' house she sits down to a simple supper with Flo and her mother during which little is said. When evening surgery is over, Dr Westbury joins them in the sitting room.

"Mum's illness is very advanced, isn't it?"

Flo's father looks at her kindly. "I'm afraid so. I think she knew that she was suffering from something serious long before she came to see me. When I gave her the diagnosis, her first words were that you should not be told about it. She was very adamant about that. She didn't want you to worry."

"I know," Holly says softly. "I only found out by accident. I wish I'd known . . . But surely she could have had more treatment than just those pills she was taking?"

"Of course," Dr Westbury replies. "I tried to persuade her to have a course of therapy at a sanatorium but she wouldn't hear of it."

"You mean she actually refused treatment?"

"Yes, she did. As I said, she didn't want to upset you or leave you on your own. She kept saying how much you mean to her. You're everything to her, you know."

Holly only nods, unable to speak.

"She also had some strange notion about not living any longer than her allotted time. There are lots of folk here in the dales who think like that. I suppose it's because they live so close to nature. They believe that there's a season for everything – plants, animals and people, too – and that when their season is over, it's time to go." He gets to his feet, suddenly looking tired and old. "My dear, it's been a long, hard day for you. I think you should try and get some rest now."

Flo takes Holly upstairs to the guest room and hugs her warmly. "I'll go with you to the hospital in the morning if you like." She turns to leave.

"Flo, don't go yet, please. There's something I have to tell you." A note of anguish in her voice makes her friend stop. She sits down on the edge of the bed and looks up at Holly, her blue eyes filled with concern.

"I think it was my fault that Mum took so ill last night."

"Your fault? Holly, how can you say that? Why should you be to blame?" Flo's expression has changed from worry to disbelief.

"I don't think it would have happened if . . ." Holly hesitates. At first the words do not come, but then they tumble from her lips as if she cannot bear to say them. "I didn't go home last night. I spent the night with Nick Ranleigh. He took me to Sands End in his car but we couldn't get back because of the snow. We spent the night together in a cottage that belongs to his family." The news which at any other time she would love to share with her dearest friend now sounds like a confession in a court of law.

Flo's eyes are round in astonishment. "Oh Holly, I know how much you've tried to hide it but anyone can see that you're in love with Nick. And does he . . ?"

"Oh Flo, he loves me too. It's so wonderful. I was so happy last night, but now . . ."

"Look here," Flo cuts in, adopting a tone not unlike that of her mother, "Dad just told you how ill your mum is. The bleeding could have started at any time. It's not your fault at all, it was nothing to do with you. You must never ever think that, and you mustn't let anything spoil what is between you and Nick! We'll go and see how she is in the morning. She may be a lot better by then."

"I'm frightened she's going to die!"

"Holly, love, nobody lives forever. We all have to go sometime but she' s getting the best possible medical care and you know what a strong nature she has. She'll pull through, I bet." She takes Holly in her arms.

"Flo, what would I do without you? But there's something else Mum told me, her last words before she went into the coma. She told me that Dad wasn't my real father. She said Dad knew, and that he loved me, but my father was – or is – somebody else! Oh, Flo, I'm so confused. I don't know what to think!"

Flo draws back amazed. She gazes intently at her friend. "Are you hurt about that? Are you mad because she didn't tell you earlier?"

"I'm not mad or hurt. How could I be? I always loved Dad, and I know he loved me."

"Do you know who your real father is?"

"No, but whoever he is, Dad will always be Dad to me. All Mum managed to say was "Philippe" – she pronounced it the French way. I don't know anyone called Philippe! How can I ever find out who I really am?"

Flo takes Holly's hands in hers. "You are you. Maybe one day you'll find out who your real father is, but that doesn't alter who you are. Remember that." She gives her a hug and whispers good-night.

When the door closes behind her friend, Holly looks around, for the first time taking in the spacious airy room with its comfortable furnishings and large sash windows, so different from the farmhouse where she has lived all her life. The fact that Tom Barton was not her father means strangely little. If anything, her feelings for him are strengthened by knowing that a poor farmer gave her so much love and shared the little he had with her. And her true father? Who is he? The question somehow does not seem important. She feels numb. She pulls back the covers and climbs into the soft bed. Then the tension of the past hours finds its release and she sobs uncontrollably into the pillow . . .

EIGHT

. . . She must have fallen into a fitful, dreamless sleep. From afar she dimly registers the shrill ringing of a telephone breaking the stillness of the night, then slippered feet padding swiftly along the carpeted landing past her room, and a thin line of light shining under the door. In the hallway downstairs she can hear muffled voices. Her fears are confirmed when the returning footsteps stop outside her bedroom and a gentle tap makes her fumble hastily for the switch of the bedside lamp.

Mrs Westbury appears in the doorway, her stout figure swathed in pink candlewick. Smelling softly of talcum powder, she lowers herself to sit on the edge of Holly's bed.

"I'm so sorry, my dear. That was the hospital ringing just now. They say your mother has taken a turn for the worse. She's not in any pain, but it seems there's nothing more they can do. I'm afraid she's sinking fast. They think you should come. I'll drive you over there at once, my dear."

Holly dresses in a trance, pulling on one garment after another. The biting cold air as they get out of the car at the hospital makes her briefly aware of her surroundings, but when she has been shepherded inside and led to her mother's room, unreality descends again. After insisting that Mrs Westbury return home, she sits alone beside her mother's unconscious form, holding her hand, watching as her life slips away. At some time in the early hours of the morning her mother's breathing becomes shallower and irregular. Then it stops, and Elizabeth Barton passes from life into death as peacefully and undramatically as she has lived.

Holly finds herself in the waiting-room again while the nurses unplug the machines that have failed to keep her mother alive. After all the apparatus of death has been removed, she will go back in and say good-bye. She wants to remember her at peace, not fighting a losing battle to live. When the door opens she looks up, expecting a nurse to enter with yet another offer of tea, but it is Nick. She flies into his arms.

"Holly, why didn't you call me? I've only just heard you're here. I would have come with you. How's your mum?"

She looks up into his face through her tears. "Oh Nick, she's gone. She died just a few minutes ago."

He says none of the usual words of sympathy or comfort but just holds her tightly, closely, as if he never wants to let her go, as if in doing so he can draw her grief into his own body.

When the nurse returns they are still standing in each other's arms, and hand in hand they go into the room where Elizabeth Barton is lying. The lines of pain and struggle have left her face; she is at peace now, as if she has fallen asleep. Holly smoothes the hair from her brow, strokes her cheek and whispers simple words of thanks and farewell.

When they leave the hospital it is still dark but already the world is beginning to come to life again. The Monday morning traffic is starting to build up as early commuters leave the still-sleeping town. Nick pulls out of the car park.

"Was it Flo who called and told you where I was?"

"Yes, and I'm glad she did. But why didn't you ring me, let me know what had happened?"

"Somehow I couldn't. I felt so awful that I wasn't there when Mum took ill. I thought it was my fault, you know, for upsetting her . . ." He wants to interrupt, frowning and shaking his head in protest, but she intervenes. "Yes, I know. I suppose it would have happened anyway. I had a talk with Flo and I'm trying to come to terms with that, but Mum's gone now and I'll never be able to explain." He takes one hand from the steering wheel and places it over hers. Briefly she tells him the news of her father.

He looks serious. "Well, if it's what you want, I'll do everything I can to help you find out who your real father is."

Holly stares out of the window, saying nothing, not knowing what she wants.

"Where do you want me to take you? Do you want to go back to the Westburys', or home?"

"Home."

The word that used to mean so much sounds empty and hollow now. There will be no one there, no one waiting for her, but it is the only place where she can bear to go.

He seems to read her thoughts. "I'll go with you. I don't want you to be there on your own. And I'll ring the Westburys and explain."

"Thank you," she says simply, and they do not speak again until the car draws up in front of Black Ridge Farm. Holly pushes the back door open, expecting to find the kitchen as cold and dark as she left it the previous day. Instead, a fire is burning in the grate, casting a warm glow in the little room and, in an armchair beside it, there is Sally, fast asleep and snoring softly. As they enter she wakes with a start and struggles to her feet.

"She's dead, Sally." Holly weeps on the little nurse's shoulder.

"There, there." Sally pats her back, comforting her like a child. "Your mum told me how bad her condition was, and I'm a nurse too, so I could see for myself. She knew she didn't have long to live. Believe me," she looks into Holly's eyes, "it was only a question of time. And in a way I'm glad . . ."

"Glad?"

"Yes, glad," Sally's voice is almost defiant. "Glad that it's over now. Over so quickly. Glad that she didn't have to suffer any longer if there was no hope of her getting better."

"I suppose you're right," Holly sighs. "Maybe it was the best for her, even if it's hard for us."

"It's always hard to lose a person you love, my dear. It's the hardest thing in the world." Sally speaks quietly, almost to herself, and Holly senses that the words have a deeper meaning than she can understand.

At Nick's and Sally's insistence Holly goes to her room to rest. She only intends to lie down for a while, but as soon as she puts her head on the pillow she falls into a heavy sleep induced by pure exhaustion. When she awakes, several hours have passed. Red puffy eyes stare back at her in the bathroom mirror. She splashes her face with cold water, brushes her teeth, drags a comb through her tangled hair and goes downstairs to find Nick and Sally at the kitchen table with plates of bacon and eggs in front of them. Her body suddenly reminds her that she has eaten almost nothing in the past twenty-four hours.

"That smells good. Any for me?"

They set a place for her between them. No one speaks while they eat. After the meal is over, Holly and Nick make Sally rest in her chair beside the fire while they do the washing-up. When they have finished, Holly takes the chair opposite Sally, where Elizabeth used to sit. Sally looks anxiously across at her, noting the pallor of her once-creamy skin and the dark circles around the formerly bright eyes.

"Sally, you and Mum talked a lot in these last weeks while she was ill. Her last word was the name 'Philippe'. Did she ever mention anybody called that?"

Sally bends down and gives all her attention to poking the embers of the fire. Knocking the white ash off a charred log, she stares at the tiny blue and orange tongues of flame licking around it. At last she speaks. "Yes, love, she did, but do you think we should begin that story now? It's been a long hard day for you. Don't you think . . . ?"

"Sally!" Holly is on her knees in front of her, as if by grasping her hands she can hold her attention. "Sally, don't you see? I've got to know more. You've got to tell me everything she said. There was something Mum wanted me to know, I'm sure, but she died before she could tell me." Her voice breaks. She pauses and wipes her eyes before she can go on. "She told me that Dad wasn't my real father." The words come out as a whisper.

Sally gives the fire another vigorous poke, then sits back in her chair, gazing into the glow. "I know," she says simply.

"You mean, Mum actually told you that?" Holly is unable to keep the hurt from mingling with the incredulity in her voice.

- 84 -

"Don't be upset, dear. Your mother and I became quite close in these last weeks. We were alone together a lot. She didn't want to burden you with – "

"Not burden me! That's exactly what Dr Westbury said! Everybody seems to have been keeping things from me all the time! Didn't you think I had a right to know? After all, I was her daughter! Why didn't she tell me?" Her anguish finds its vent in anger.

"My dear, you'll find out when you're older that there are some things that it's easier to talk about with someone of your own age, especially when that person has been through a similar experience. One day Elizabeth noticed that I'd been crying. It was the anniversary of the day William, my fiancé, and I got engaged in 1939, the year before he was killed at Dunkirk. That's how we got talking and that's when she told me."

Holly says nothing. She is beginning to realize that her mother was not the only person who had secrets.

"I think she had some sort of premonition that she was going to die soon. The next morning, while you were at work, I found her in the sitting-room sorting through all the papers in the bureau and I had the feeling that she was putting her affairs in order, though I didn't say anything at the time. And then she showed me this, and asked me to give it to you one day. "One day", she said, and we both knew which day she meant . . ."

This time it is Sally who cannot go on. She wipes her eyes with the corner of her apron before she gets up and goes over to the kitchen dresser. She opens one of the drawers and pulls out a large brown envelope. Holly's name is written in her mother's neat hand on the front.

"Your mother wanted to tell you the truth about your father when you were twenty-one – she said that you would be old enough to understand then – but if anything happened to her before then, I was to give you this." She holds out the envelope.

Holly takes it, wondering. She can feel Nick's eyes on her as she opens it. The contents slide into her lap. The document lying on the top is her birth certificate, stating that a girl, Holly, was born to Thomas Edward Barton, farmer, and his wife, Elizabeth Mary Barton, on September 2nd, 1944.

The second document is similar in size and shape. Holly unfolds it carefully to find it is her parents' marriage certificate, stating that Thomas Edward Barton, bachelor of this parish, married Elizabeth Mary Fairley, spinster, on July 18th, 1944.

She stares at the date. "There must be a mistake," she stammers. "Mum and Dad were married in 1943. When Dad was home on leave from the army."

"No, my dear," Sally interjects gently. "There isn't any mistake."

"But that must mean . . . that Mum was – " somehow she cannot bring herself to use the word 'pregnant' – "was expecting me when she and Dad got married." She turns to face Sally. "But she told me that Dad knew he wasn't my father! Did she marry him knowing she was expecting another man's child?"

"Take a look at the other papers first."

Holly stares at the small heap in her lap. She picks up a small photograph. It has faded over the years, the edges are roughened and it is creased as though it has been carried in a purse or pocket for a long time. It is a black-and-white studio portrait of young man with thick dark hair and classical features, a strong jaw line and a straight nose, wearing a shirt that is open at the neck. It is a formal pose with him looking sidewards past the camera, but the photographer's efforts to give him a distinguished air are belied by the curve of his lips and the sparkle of laughter in his eyes. Holly turns it over. On the back there is the stamp of a London photographer and the words, *'Pour Elizabeth – Philippe'*.

Holly is looking at the face of her father.

When she raises her eyes, Sally only nods, indicating that she should go on. The last item in her lap is a thick sheet of paper. She picks it up and turns it over. It is a pen-and-ink sketch that has been folded to fit into an envelope. She holds it closer to the light. It shows a woodland glade with trees overhanging a brook. On the bank a young woman is lying on her back, perfectly relaxed, the folds of her summer dress moulding her slim figure, one arm behind her head. She is watching the artist, a slight smile playing on her lips. It is her mother, there is no doubt. The artist – and Holly's instincts tell her that it can only have been a man – has managed to convey all the longing and sensuality of love with a few strokes of his pen. At the bottom there are the initials P. de V. One look at the expression in her mother's eyes tells her that the artist can only have been Philippe. Was this artist, Philippe, her father?

Sally seems to have heard her unasked question.

"Elizabeth told me that Philippe was the love of her life and the father of her child."

Holly stares at the sketch, her thoughts racing. "But Sally, she must have told you more than that! Who was he? What happened to him? Why didn't they marry? Why did she marry Dad instead?" So many questions, but where are the answers?

"I'm afraid I don't know any more about him, my dear. She only told me that his name was Philippe. He was French – from Paris she said – and he was an artist. They met in London during the war when your mother was serving in the Women's Auxiliary Air Force."

Suddenly Holly knows why her mother always refused to talk about her experiences in the war years. It was the one time in her life when she left the dale. Like many people, she experienced more in those few years than in all the years that followed or went before, yet she never spoke of them. Holly has always imagined that this was because of the horrors she witnessed during the Blitz. Only now does she realize that her mother's suffering was more personal.

"But why did he leave her? Surely he didn't abandon her when she was expecting a baby? He couldn't have! Not if they loved each other so much!"

Sally draws a deep breath before she speaks. "He never found out. I'm sorry to have to tell you this, Holly, but he suddenly broke off their affair. Elizabeth had been posted to an airfield in Devon. She wrote to him with the news of her pregnancy but he didn't reply. All her letters were returned unopened. She never heard from him again."

Holly is overwhelmed by a sense of loss. Seeing the tears well in her eyes, Nick takes her in his arms. Huge sobs shake her body. It is as if she has lost her father once more, but this time she does not even have any memories to cling to.

"So what did Mum do?" she asks Sally at last.

"What could she do? She did the only thing she could do – she came home, back to the dale. Of course she couldn't keep her pregnancy a secret for long. Her own mother had died at the beginning of the war, her father was absolutely furious and disowned her, and the only person she could turn to was Tom."

"Dad?"

"Yes. They had been friends since their school days. He had always loved her and still did. There was no chance of her getting a job to support herself and her child and there weren't all the social benefits then that there are nowadays. But above all, you've got to remember that being an unmarried mother was a fate worse than death in those times. There was no question of getting rid of the baby. She told me she never even considered that. It was her child and Philippe's, she said. Tom offered to stand by her. He loved her, he could offer her a home and he promised to bring up her baby as if it were his own. So, even knowing she could never love him as she had loved Philippe, she accepted."

"But she and Dad were always so happy together!"

"There are different kinds of happiness, dear. Tom was a kind man, a good husband and a loving father, and she came to love him deeply too, just in a different way. And I know they both loved you more than anything else on earth."

"I know they did." Holly's eyes are again misty with tears. She brushes them away with the back of her hand.

Sally is gathering up her bags and her coat. "I'll have to be getting home now. I'll be back first thing in the morning, love." She gives Holly a hug, says good bye to Nick and leaves them alone together.

"May I stay? I don't want to leave you alone, not after all

you've been through today," he whispers as he takes her in his arms again. He strokes her hair. "Just for tonight."

"Yes, don't go. Stay with me, please." He kisses her lips tenderly before she speaks again. "But what will happen about your lectures? You really should have gone back yesterday, shouldn't you?"

He shakes his head, his grey eyes never leaving hers. "This is more important. If I leave for London very early in the morning I'll make it by the afternoon."

They know that the night to come will be very different from the passionate hours they spent in the old cottage. Arms entwined, they slowly climb the stairs.

NINE

Paris, Spring 1967

How many times had she stood at her window in the early hours of the morning, unable to sleep, gazing at the city of Paris spread out before her, wondering where her father might be? At that very moment he might be only minutes away, unaware that she was looking for him, unaware that she even existed. When she had come to France two years ago, she had so hoped that she would find him, a hope that had been dashed within weeks. There were so many Philippe de Vs in the Parisian telephone book. Her endless tours of the many art galleries had led to nothing. All the dealers to whom she had shown the sketch of Elizabeth had agreed that it had been carried out by a very talented artist, but one with whose work they were not familiar.

Holly took the drawing from the drawer of her bedside table, still in the brown envelope with her mother's handwriting on the front. She pulled it out and studied it for the thousandth time. Surely there must be a clue somewhere. Then her eyes fell on her little alarm clock; it was nine o'clock, the time when she went to Arlette's boudoir to discuss the day's business. With a sigh she slid the sketch into the envelope again and pushed it back into the drawer, as if in doing so she could trap her disappointment inside as well.

Although she did her best to hide her emotions, Arlette was quick to notice the pallor of her face and the dark shadows beneath her eyes. "You have been having too many late nights, my dear," she admonished gently. "That nephew of mine has been overtiring you, I fear." She patted the bed, motioned Holly to sit down beside her and took off her reading glasses. Her voice dropped, taking on a more serious note.

"Ma chère, during these last few days I have been

wondering if I should not warn you. Julien is – how one says? – très charmant. He is good-looking and very rich. He has inherited vast properties, vineyards and investments on the Bourse, but . . ." She paused and looked into Holly's eyes. Her voice softened. "I do not want you to be hurt, my dear. Julien takes after his father, my husband's brother-in-law. Such men do not make a woman happy. They like to amuse themselves but their feelings do not go deep. They love the company and admiration of young and beautiful women but they do not give their hearts."

Holly smiled at the older woman. "Don't worry, madame. I'm not in love with Julien," she said shyly. "It's like a dream here, a wonderful dream, and one day I'll wake up." She smiled. "But until that day comes, I'm learning all I can –and enjoying every minute!"

"Then let's get on with today's lesson." Arlette's worried expression relaxed. She replaced her reading glasses and picked up an opened letter from her lap. "Something new for you, chérie! An assignment all on your own! As you know, I have to go to our Italian office next week but we have decided to bring forward a special feature on knitwear for the magazine. I cannot possibly go to Milan and manage the photo shoot for the knitwear as well. So, ma chère, I shall have to go to Italy on my own and I'd like you to take over for me here. Jean-Pierre Fôret is doing the photography. He knows exactly what we need for the feature. The models are already booked and the location is arranged, so there's not a lot left to do except to see it through. Do you think you could cover the assignment for me?"

"Oh, madame!" Holly was breathless with excitement. "I'd love to. If you think I'm up to it."

"Call me Arlette, please. After all, we are colleagues now." She smiled at her young protégée reassuringly. "I'd have taken you along to ask your opinion anyway, so I'm sure you'll be fine. Don't worry. Jean-Pierre is an old fox. He knows what to do. The knitwear is cashmere so it requires a classic setting for it to look perfect. I made the arrangements for the location myself."

"Yes, I remember. It's the Château d'Ivry, isn't it? I know

about it but I've no idea exactly where the château is."

"It is about 150 kilometres south-west of Paris, on the Loire. Not one of the famous châteaux – it's only small and not open to the public. But it's very beautiful. The Vicomtesse d'Ivry still lives there. She's a distant relation of my late husband – that's how I was able to arrange the session. She doesn't normally allow strangers onto her property but I was able – how you English say? – to pull a few strings."

"So we'll only be there for the day?"

"Yes. If you get off to an early start, you shouldn't have any problems. Only two models and six or seven shots are needed for the feature. The light is good at this time of year and since you'll be shooting indoors, you won't have any trouble with the weather either."

"I'm looking forward to it." Holly looked earnest. "I'll do my best, Arlette," she added shyly, using her name for the first time.

"I have no worries on that score," the Frenchwoman smiled. "Now if I could be just as sure of my success in Milan without you, I would have no worries at all!"

The intervening days passed quickly. On the evening of her departure Arlette invited Comte Maurice and Julien to join her and Holly for an intimate souper à quatre in her apartment before she boarded the sleeper for Milan. Any fears that Holly might have had on meeting Julien again proved to be unfounded. If anything, her rejection of him after their visit to the theatre seemed to have heightened his interest in her, and he was more charming and attentive than ever. Deciding that she had been acting like a silly schoolgirl, Holly enjoyed his company. Julien revealed himself to have a wicked sense of humour and his clever parodies of well-known figures in French public life, most of whom Holly was able to recognize, had them all laughing and joking until Arlette regretfully rose to take her car to the station, bringing the evening to a close.

The following morning, the day of her first solo assignment, Holly awoke feeling apprehensive. Unable to face breakfast, she was waiting nervously outside when the minibus arrived to pick her up. Immediately she was struck by the relaxed mood of its occupants; what for her was an exciting challenge was daily routine for them.

The peaceful and pleasant countryside of the Loire valley with its thick woodlands and sleepy villages unveiled itself before her eyes through the blue haze of the Gauloises which Jean-Pierre was chain-smoking behind the wheel. The two models, Carmen and Britt, a tall raven-haired Venezuelan and an even lankier Swedish blonde, were sitting in the back with Pia, the Italian hairstylist and visagist, conversing in that particular brand of American-English which had become the mother tongue of their profession. None of the three bothered even to glance at the passing scenery; they had seen locations like this a thousand times before.

Holly marvelled at the density of the forests, their largely deciduous trees already a fresh green. Spring was advancing rapidly. Unlike the cultivated woods of England, these forests were a tumble of natural vegetation. Dead branches and trunks uprooted by long-gone storms had been left to rot where they had fallen. Mistletoe and ivy entwined themselves from bough to bough, creating an impenetrable tangle through which the rays of the morning sun filtered into mossy glades where masses of tiny white wood anemones gleamed like a soft carpet of snow.

They rounded a bend in the road and Holly caught her breath in disbelief. Pinnacles, turrets and towers rose suddenly out of the depths of the forest ahead. Like a fairytale castle the château seemed to emerge from the fifteenth century. As they approached, the trees parted to reveal a wide carriageway lined with rhododendrons in full bloom. The lushness of the extravagant pink, white, red and purple blooms was almost tropical. At the end of the drive huge, age-old iron gates had been flung back, giving access to a gravelled courtyard.

Jean-Pierre stopped the bus in front of a broad flight of

worn stone steps and without further ado began unloading his cameras and lighting equipment. Carmen, Britt and Pia continued their conversation, seemingly unaware of their arrival. Holly, acutely conscious of being in charge of the whole operation, tried to assume an air of self-assurance which she did not feel, whilst wondering what to do first. Her problem was solved by an elderly white-haired gentleman who somewhat unsteadily descended the steps to greet them.

Since he nodded courteously but did not attempt to shake her hand, Holly assumed that he must be a butler or other sort of house servant, a fact which was borne out by the formal manner of his French greeting. "Mademoiselle Barton? Madame La Vicomtesse d'Ivry has asked me to present her compliments to you and assure you of the co-operation of her staff in the successful completion of your tasks."

Holly nodded in acknowledgement, and summoning all her linguistic resources, begged him in similar style to convey her cordial thanks to his mistress.

In the wake of the ancient retainer, they mounted the steps to enter a large, flag-stoned hall. Despite the bright sunshine outside and huge logs burning in the two great fireplaces at opposite ends of the room, Holly shivered at the chill which at once fell upon them. On an upper floor, a bedroom which seemed even colder had been placed at their disposal so that the models could change. It was clearly not used by the inhabitants of the house. Holly unpacked the exquisite collection of Italian knitwear and laid it out on the threadbare silk counterpane of the huge oak bed. Together with a vast wooden chest placed against one of the walls, this made up the only furniture in the chamber. Long, dusty green hangings lined the floor-length windows which overlooked an empty inner courtyard. Having found a bathroom which actually possessed a wall socket where they could plug in their electric rollers, Britt and Carmen returned giggling and rolling their eyes in horror at the antiquated plumbing.

Leaving Pia to style the girls' hair and apply their make-up, Holly went downstairs to where Jean-Pierre was surveying the merits of their location. The hall with its magnificent staircase, tall windows, elaborate fireplaces and walls thickly hung with tapestries, seemed an excellent setting despite the cold. Holly began to relax as Jean-Pierre, light-meter in hand, began taking readings to see where they should place the models. "Better start at the windows as long as the light holds," he muttered through his cigarette. "It's nearly twelve already."

The hours flew past. Britt and Carmen were true professionals. Pia had swept up their long hair and applied a superb makeup which brought out Britt's cool Nordic beauty and underlined Carmen's smouldering Latin sensuality. The contrast was stunning. Both styles, though so different, were absolutely classic and made the cashmere knitwear look luxurious, exclusive and utterly feminine. The two girls' chatter and laughter had ceased immediately when work began. On Holly's directions they gazed wistfully out of the windows, relaxed elegantly at the foot of the carved staircase, leaned languidly against the heavy panelled doors.

As the afternoon light began to fade, Jean-Pierre was engaged in the last, most demanding shots. Only the evening knitwear still had to be photographed. Wearing fine, low-cut black and white tops delicately embroidered with tiny beads of jet and pearls respectively, Carmen and Britt posed gracefully at the fireplace in its flickering light.

The room seemed even colder than it had been that morning. The air was thick with the smoke of Jean-Pierre's numerous Gauloises. Holly's head was aching and she was beginning to feel acutely conscious of the fact that she had not eaten that day, yet the models seemed as cool and fresh as ever. Not for the first time, Holly admired the stamina and professionalism of these girls who were generally considered to earn exorbitant fees for being no more than walking clotheshorses. Nor did she fail to notice that their hostess, who had not appeared at all, had neglected to offer them any sort of refreshment. Jean-Pierre laughed grimly when she commented on this fact. "What do you expect, ma petite? Everyone thinks this is an easy job. It is – how you say so charmingly in English? – money for old rope, n'est-ce pas?"

Two more reels of film and the shots were taken. Half an hour to pack, two hours to drive back to the city, Holly reflected, and then she could climb into a hot tub and relax. She heaved a sigh of anticipation mixed with relief. It made a difference being on her own, rather than trotting round after Arlette taking notes. Tomorrow she could visit Jean–Pierre at his studio and see the photographs as he developed them. She was already looking forward to helping him choose which ones would appear in the magazine. As Jean–Pierre stacked his equipment in the back of the minibus, she felt that her first solo assignment had been a success.

Pia, Carmen and Britt had resumed their conversation of the morning in the back when Holly climbed wearily into the passenger seat. Jean-Pierre switched on the head-lamps and turned the ignition key. The engine spluttered unconvincingly into life and died away again almost at once. Jean-Pierre uttered a violent Gallic curse and tried again. This time the engine barely responded and an ominous silence descended. After several further unsuccessful attempts, the following minutes were spent with five heads anxiously peering under the bonnet of the ancient vehicle.

"It seems to be the battery. It needs recharging. Merde! Why do I always get the old vans?" Jean-Pierre slammed the lid down and ground the butt of his last Gauloise ferociously into the ground with the heel of one of his Chelsea boots.

Holly felt that she should take charge. "It's no good," she announced, summoning up her last reserves of energy in an effort to sound confident, "we're going to need help to get this thing started."

Like an answer to their prayers, the specks of two headlamps appeared at that moment at the far end of the carriageway. In the falling darkness they gradually grew larger and a Rolls Royce Silver Shadow purred into the courtyard and stopped behind them. A uniformed chauffeur jumped out and strode round to the other side of the car where he deferentially opened the door. An elderly lady emerged from its depths. She was a tiny, almost wizened person and, despite the mild weather, dressed in tweeds and furs. Holly realized that this could only be the Vicomtesse d'Ivry, which was fortunate since the woman did not deem it necessary to introduce herself to her visitors.

"Bonsoir, mademoiselle. You must be Mademoiselle Barton, n'est-ce pas? I am delighted to meet you. How is my dear friend and cousin, Madame de Châtigny? I hope your day's work has been to your satisfaction?" Holly was uncertain whether she spoke English out of courtesy to her guests or simply assumed that these foreigners would not have sufficient command of her own language. Speaking in English, Holly answered both questions before venturing to explain their current predicament.

"Mais il n'y a pas de problème – there is no problem. Charles here will help you." She motioned airily to the chauffeur, who sprang to attention. Madame la Vicomtesse was clearly a person who was used to having her orders obeyed. "And until your vehicle is ready, please do step inside again. You cannot wait here in this damp evening air, so dangerous for the bronchial passages. I trust you have been well looked after by my staff? Was the luncheon to your taste?"

Following her up the steps into the house again, Holly interrupted the flow of words to point out that they had not, in fact, been offered any food at all. The Vicomtesse stopped and turned to face her, her eyes wide with horror at this appalling breech of her creed of hospitality. On his appearance the butler was met by a torrent of rapid French, punctuated with violent gestures to which he had neither the courage nor the opportunity to reply.

Inside the château their hostess peeled off her furs. A housemaid rushed to remove them along with the visitors' coats, and they were soon seated at the fire in the hall once more. This time, solicitous enquiries were made whether they wished to eat and drink. The result was that China tea was served in thin porcelain cups, so pale that it looked and tasted like perfumed water, accompanied by some very dry wafers. "And of course you will all be my guests at dinner," their hostess announced. The invitation was issued as a statement of fact rather than a question and their polite refusals went unheeded at first, but eventually it became clear that Carmen, Britt and Pia preferred to return to the city, pleading bookings that demanded them to be at work very early the next morning, though Holly strongly suspected that they all had dates for the evening. Charles was promptly summoned to drive the three women in the Rolls to the nearest railway station and from there they could catch the train to Paris.

Holly envied them greatly, all the more so when the chauffeur announced that the minibus not only had a flat battery but also an ignition fault which he was unable to correct. He had already rung the nearest garage and someone was coming to tow the bus away for repairs. Unwilling to take his valuable photographic equipment or the clothes they had been modelling on such an expedition, Jean-Pierre unloaded them all again and, leaving everything with Holly, departed with the promise to pick her up as soon as the bus had been repaired.

"And so, my dear mademoiselle, you will do me the honour of dining with me at eight. That will give me the opportunity not only of hearing all the news about ma chère Madame de Châtigny but also of compensating for the lack of hospitality which my servants have so regrettably shown towards you and your colleagues today."

Holly wondered where she could summon the strength to spend an evening engaged in such stilted conversation after the exhausting day she had spent. When her hostess offered her the chance of freshening up before dinner, she thankfully accepted and soon found herself once again in the upstairs room, which this time seemed even colder and emptier than before. She dropped wearily onto the bed and tried to relax, not daring to close her eyes for fear that she should fall asleep and cause offence by not appearing punctually at dinner. She felt that she owed it to Arlette to be polite and friendly.

It was shortly before eight o'clock when Holly rose and washed her face in the adjoining bathroom. She had neither a change of clothes nor fresh make-up, so she just combed her hair and applied a touch of lipstick. Then she took a deep breath and went downstairs to take up the daunting invitation to dine with this formidable lady.

TEN

Dinner was served in the vast banqueting hall. Two places had been laid at the long table of massive mahogany, but Holly got the impression that the vicomtesse always dined there even when alone, and felt as if she had stepped into the pages of a nineteenth-century novel. She was almost expecting Miss Havisham to appear in her wedding gown, but when the viscomtesse entered the room she was wearing a long black dress. She sat down, motioning Holly to do likewise. The white-gloved butler served decanted wines, while an elderly maidservant waited on the two diners.

It was a French dîner in the classic tradition: the soup, a thin julienne of celery and carrots, was followed by a loup de mer, a white fish which the butler deftly filleted at the table, succeeded by a gigot of spring lamb. A green salad and cheeses followed, then a Charlotte russe as dessert, and finally fruit. There was far more food than they could possibly have eaten, even with hearty appetites. In fact, Holly reflected, her whole party could scarcely have managed it all. She herself was hungry and ate with relish, but the Vicomtesse d'Ivry did little more than taste each dish as it was placed before her. Having grown up in an environment in which food had not been plentiful and was certainly never wasted, Holly found herself wondering what would happen to the leftovers. She feared they would be thrown away.

Conversation progressed amicably during the meal as Holly answered her hostess's questions about Arlette – her health, her state of mind following the tragic loss of her husband and daughter, her professional life and her position in Parisian society. The vicomtesse made it clear, however, that she did not think it right that a woman of Arlette de Châtigny's social standing should work at all. Courtesy and tiredness prevented

Holly from contradicting these views and trying to explain how much Arlette's profession meant to her. Although Arlette could certainly have managed financially without working, since her husband had left her well-provided for and she came from a wealthy background, Holly knew that Arlette's job was far more to her than mere money. Using her creative talent offered her greater pleasure and fulfilment than the Parisian social whirl. Above all, her work had given her life a new purpose and meaning after the death of her loved ones.

Holly doubted greatly whether the vicomtesse would have understood; there was a haughtiness and disdain in her manner which made Holly refrain from even attempting to argue with her. She did not imagine that the old lady could ever have suffered as Arlette had done. She seemed to have been born to a life of wealth and ease, a life spent far away from the cares of the real world, hidden in a fairytale castle with servants on call to carry out her every wish. Holly found it hard to believe that this old woman with the severe lines on her proud features had once been young. Had she ever loved or been loved?

As the evening progressed, the conversation became more and more one-sided. The monotonous voice at the far end of the table launched into a monologue on the evils of the modern world. When her eyelids began to droop, Holly pinched her arm to keep herself awake. Though she had been careful only to taste each vintage as it was served, the wine was starting to take its toll. She felt as if a thick hedge was growing up around the castle and its châtelaine, distancing them from the present day, drawing them all down into a deep, deep slumber . . .

The voice had suddenly ceased speaking. Abruptly Holly looked down to the far end of the table and realized that her hostess had risen to her feet, announcing that coffee would be taken in the salon. Perhaps a dose of caffeine would give her the strength she needed to see the evening to its close. The butler opened the doors for them to pass into the drawing room, where his mistress dismissed him, announcing that she would serve the coffee herself.

The vicomtesse directed Holly to take one of a pair of armchairs directly in front of the fire, and set about pouring steaming black liquid from a silver pot. The heavy aroma of mocha pervaded the room. Feeling warmer and more comfortable than she had done all day, Holly accepted the delicate cup and saucer that her hostess handed to her and turned to place it on a pedestal table at her side. As she did so, she noticed a large photograph there, prominently displayed in an ornate silver frame. She recognized the former French president, General Charles de Gaulle, in his grey military uniform. The portrait, taken when he was younger and before he had come to political power, was signed with a hand-written dedication. Desperate for a topic of conversation, Holly seized the opportunity.

"I see you have a photograph of de Gaulle, madame. Is the general linked to your family in any way?"

"Ah, mademoiselle," the vicomtesse's proud face creased into the semblance of a smile. "Le Général! What a fine soldier, a great leader of our Grande Nation! The portrait was personally presented by the general to my eldest son, Auguste, the present vicomte, in 1945."

Holly searched her mind for snippets of information from conversations she had heard at Arlette's dinner parties. "After the occupation of France at the beginning of the war, de Gaulle refused to cooperate with the Germans and fled to London, didn't he?"

The old lady's retort was prompt and sharp. "Cooperate? Collaborate! The politicians of the Vichy regime who capitulated to the Nazis were traitors, mademoiselle! When de Gaulle made his famous speech in London in June 1940 rallying the French troops, Auguste was one of the sons of France's noble families who rushed to join him there, together with many brave men from our colonies overseas. That was how the Free French movement was founded."

An idea was starting to form in Holly's mind, like a tiny spark which, if nurtured, she hoped might burst into flame. She needed to know if French troops had been stationed in London in 1944. Choosing her words carefully she asked, "Did your son stay in London throughout the war, madame?"

The answer was not as she had hoped. "Of course not! When de Gaulle moved his headquarters to Algiers in 1943, Auguste went with him. He served in North Africa and marched at the head of the Second Armoured Division of the Free French army when the city of Paris was liberated from the Germans in 1944."

"So there weren't any Free French in London after 1943?" Holly's voice sounded thin and anguished.

"Oh, I daresay there may have been a few. London was important for de Gaulle, though his relations with Churchill were always strained. Churchill never really acknowledged what a great leader de Gaulle . . ."

The rambling voice continued and then stopped. The vicomtesse was staring into the fire, lost in her thoughts of the past. Trembling, Holly managed to put down her cup without spilling any coffee. Seconds passed in which only the ticking of the clock could be heard. Her thoughts were racing. Maybe there had been Free French troops still serving in London in 1944! London was where her mother had met Philippe. They had met during the war, so perhaps her father had been in uniform, too. Why had she not thought of that before! As a regular French serviceman he would have been posted in France or North Africa or taken prisoner by the Germans, unless – the chance was slight but it was still a chance – unless he too had refused to serve under the Vichy regime and had fled to join de Gaulle, in which case he might still have been in London in 1944.

Only minutes later, to Holly's intense relief, the butler announced Jean-Pierre's return. The mini-bus was repaired and Holly was able to take her leave. During the drive back to Paris she kept her eyes closed, praying that Jean-Pierre would think she had fallen asleep. She could not bear to talk; she had to think. She had to find out if a Philippe de V. had been serving with the Free French in London in 1944.

The next morning Holly rose late after a night in which she had slept little. Arlette was still in Milan. She wanted to go to Jean-Pierre's studio to discuss the previous day's photos, but he had firmly informed her that, except when out on a shoot, the working day did not begin for him before noon. Holly took her coffee into Arlette's study and sat down at the desk, though her mind was not on work. The vicomtesse's words kept echoing in her brain. How could she find out more?

She toyed with the thought of going to a public library to look up the history of the Free French, but rejected the idea as it would not provide the information she wanted. She needed access to the military records; somewhere there must be lists of names and addresses of those who had served. Then her eye fell on the telephone. Of course! Why had she not thought of him before? Comte Maurice de Villiers, Arlette's friend. The aristocratic banker had contacts in the highest, most influential circles of French society not only by birth but also by profession. He had always been kind and helpful towards her. She found his number and dialled hopefully.

"Holly! Bonjour, ma petite! How nice to hear from you." His voice took on a sudden note of panic. "What's the matter? Is Arlette alright? Has something happened?"

"No, Maurice, not at all, everything's fine," Holly was quick to reassure him. If she had not guessed long ago that Maurice was in love with Arlette, she would have recognized it now. "This has nothing to do with Arlette. I'm calling on a personal matter, something I need to know quite urgently. Perhaps you can help me."

"Of course, ma chère Holly. What can I do for you?" His voice was calm and courteous again.

"Maurice, do you know where I can trace someone who may have been serving with the Free French in London in 1944?

If Maurice was surprised by her request he did not show it. He thought for a moment. "1944," he murmured. "There can't have been many in London then. Most of them would have left in 1943. But I believe that a skeleton staff stayed on. London was a very important stronghold for de Gaulle. Who is it you want to trace?"

Holly took a deep breath. "All I have to go on is that his first name was Philippe and his family name began de V. He was serving in London in 1944."

"And you want me to track him down for you?" He was too discreet to inquire about her motives and she did not offer to explain.

"Please, Maurice. That would be wonderful. And anything else you can find out about the family. It's really important to me."

"Of course, my dear. It shouldn't be too difficult. I'll see what I can do and ring you back this evening."

Holly thanked him and rang off. She looked at her watch. It was nearly eleven. There was no point in trying to concentrate on any work. Besides, it was a beautiful spring day. If she set off now, she could walk along the banks of the Seine to Jean-Pierre's studio and be there at twelve.

The photographs were hanging in the darkroom to dry when she arrived. Jean-Pierre had clearly exaggerated his laziness. He must have been working all morning, she noted, judging by the overflowing ashtray and the smoke-laden air inside the little room. As they pored over the photos together, Holly listened with interest to his comments. The photos she herself would have chosen were not, in his eyes, the best. It was not simply the content, lighting and composition of a shot that mattered, it was more the atmosphere that a photo evoked. She had often heard talk of the 'art' of photography but it was only now that she began to understand exactly where the art lay.

During the afternoon they spent together Holly learned a great deal, and by the time they parted she saw Jean-Pierre as an artist, not just the brilliant photographer he so clearly was.

It was early evening when she returned to the apartment where Madame Tourbie had provided a simple meal for her.

Holly ate quickly and went to sit at Arlette's desk. When the phone rang shortly before nine, she pounced on it.

"Maurice?"

"Hey, who's Maurice? Another of your handsome men? What's happened to the gorgeous Julien?" A cheery English and very familiar voice met her ears.

"Flo! How great to hear from you! I didn't expect . . ."

"Obviously not," her friend remarked dryly. "It's only me. Sorry to disappoint you!"

"Don't be stupid," Holly laughed. "It's lovely to hear from you. How are things in England?" Her voice took on a touch of anxiety. Continental phone calls were so expensive that Flo did not normally ring her. There must be some reason. Something must have happened.

Flo's next words confirmed her fears. "Look, love, I'm afraid I've got some bad news. It's Sally. She died last night."

Holly fell silent. Sally, the bustling little nurse with her bobbing curls and boundless energy who had cared for her mother during the long weeks before she died – now she had gone too.

"I'm sorry," she said simply. She had known that Sally had been terminally ill, but even so, the news was a shock.

"Perhaps it's for the best," Flo said gently. "The cancer was so far gone when it was discovered that there was no hope she would get better, so at least she didn't have to suffer long. You'd never have known how poorly she was if you had seen her. She was busy helping other people right up to the end."

"How typical of Sally!" Holly smiled at the recollection. "I suppose there'll be a big funeral, won't there? Everybody knew and loved her."

"Yes, but she said she didn't want any flowers. She's asked people to donate money to the children's ward at the hospital."

"That's just like her. Sally all over." They talked on for several minutes before Holly changed the subject.

"There was something in your last letter, Flo, something I think you should be telling me about." She could practically see

Flo blushing at the other end. "What about that date you were going on with Mike? How was it? What happened? Come on, if you can't tell your best friend your secrets, who can you tell?"

"Oh Holly – ," Flo began, and then the words came tumbling out. It was as if all the feelings for Mike, which she had kept bottled up since their schooldays, had suddenly been released. Mike was so wonderful, so sweet, so caring. She was the luckiest girl in the world.

"I'm so happy for you, Flo. I've always thought that you two were just meant for each other."

"Well, Mike's still at agricultural college because he's going to take over his dad's farm one day, but we try to see each other as often as we can. But what about you, Holly? Oh, I do so envy you sometimes – living in Paris, going to fashion shows, dating gorgeous men!"

"It's fun. Another world from Yorkshire." For a moment she was tempted to tell Flo about her efforts to trace her father, but decided against it. She could easily be mistaken and Maurice's enquiries might lead to nothing. Instead she told her friend about some of the places to which Julien had taken her.

"It all sounds so utterly, utterly romantic!" Although Flo sighed wistfully, Holly knew she would never want to change places with her. "Keep me posted, especially on any developments regarding Julien!" Flo told her as they said their good-byes, with promises to write.

Holly sat unmoving at Arlette's desk. She thought of her own words, just spoken: "If you can't tell your best friend your secrets, who can you tell?" How true they were. Only Flo, her dearest friend, knew the secret she kept hidden in her heart.

She was jolted out of her thoughts when the phone rang again. This time it was Maurice. He came straight to the point.

"There was a Captain Philippe de Valmont serving with the Free French in London in 1944. I did a bit of research on the family, Holly. Genealogy has always been a hobby of mine. The Valmonts are one of France's oldest and most noble families. The title of Chevalier was bestowed on the first Valmont by King

Henry of Navarre for saving his life on the battlefield in the sixteenth century. The Château de Valmont is situated near Bordeaux and has a small but excellent vineyard, but during the Great Depression in the early thirties, Guy de Valmont, Philippe's father, was forced to sell off the entire estate to pay death duties, so the family moved to Paris. Then Philippe, their only child, the son and heir, was killed in London. A tragic story really."

A hand of ice had gripped her heart. She was in freefall, plunging from joy to despair in the space of a few seconds. She forced herself to speak. She had to know more.

"How did he die? What happened?"

"I asked that question too, but my contact didn't know."

"And are any members of the family still alive?" She held her breath.

An agonizing pause followed. Maurice seemed to be checking his notes. "As far as I could find out, the only surviving member of that branch of the Valmont family is the father, Guy de Valmont. He must be in his seventies now. He's still living here in Paris at 22, rue du Vieux Moulin – that's somewhere in the sixteenth arrondissement, near the Bois de Boulogne."

Holly managed to note the address, thank Maurice and ring off before bursting into tears. She let her head fall onto her arms and huge sobs racked her body.

Had she found her father at last, only to lose him in the same instant? All her life she had lost everyone and everything she ever loved. Once again she felt utterly alone . . .

ELEVEN

North Yorkshire, March 1963

. . . On a late winter's day that holds the promise of spring, she is standing at her mother's grave, while Elizabeth Barton is buried as quietly and unpretentiously as she lived. The last vestiges of snow in the churchyard nestling around St Nicholas' church are melting in the rays of the noonday sunlight. The adjacent black ruins of the ancient priory stand outlined against a sky washed with aquarelle blue, and beyond the Applegarth the hills rising to the moors are tinged with the early green of larch trees. Yet when the moment comes to lower the coffin into the waiting earth, none of nature's signs of reincarnation can soften the act, or in any way lessen the finality of the parting. Holly turns from the grave so dazed with grief that she cannot even cry.

In the Victorian tradition of Yorkshire families, a wake is held afterwards for those who have attended the ceremony. In the past Holly has found the idea of a funeral tea off-putting, but now she knows that her mother would have wished to extend hospitality to everyone who has come to bid her farewell. She is glad that those who have known and cared for Elizabeth are to be with her a little longer, postponing the moment when she will be alone.

The Westburys suggested a café meal, even offering to cover the expenses, but Holly insisted that everyone should come to the farmhouse. She has gratefully accepted the plentiful offers of home-made cakes, scones and freshly-cut sandwiches. Looking around the kitchen and the front sitting-room, she is moved to see how many have come to pay Elizabeth their last respects, despite the quiet life she led. It comforts her to hear so many voices affectionately praising her in their soft Yorkshire accents.

When the last of the guests have gone, Holly is left with

Flo, Mrs Westbury and Sally amid piles of washing-up. "Come back with us, my dear," Flo's mother urges. "Come and stay with us for a while. This is no place for you to be on your own. We've got plenty of room, and my husband and I . . ."

"Yes, Holly. Please," Flo breaks in eagerly. "Come to our house. I can't bear to think of you all alone here."

"You're so kind, both of you. I haven't made up my mind yet, but somehow I just can't bear to leave the farm standing empty."

"Look, love." Sally removes the dishcloth from Holly's hands and makes her sit down at the fireside with a cup of strong tea. "For a start, drink this and eat that buttered scone. I've been watching you and you haven't had a drink or a thing to eat all day. You can't go on like that." She stands over Holly and waits until she has bitten into the scone before she speaks again. "And this is your home, so you can stay here as long as you want. As for tonight, I'm staying with you."

Taking over Holly's place at the sink, she plunges her hands into the washing-up bowl and hands Mrs Westbury a dripping plate to dry. The doctor's wife opens her mouth in contradiction but the bright blue eyes and resolute figure before her make her change her mind and she shuts it again without a word.

In the evening when they are alone at last, Holly and Sally take their usual places in front of the fire.

"The funeral was exactly as Mum would have liked it. Nothing fancy, just nice." Holly sighs. "Thanks for staying with me tonight, Sally."

"Well, I didn't want you being here on your own."

"Nick wanted to stay for the funeral but I told him not to. He missed so many lectures last week because of me." They sit in silence for a while, each lost in her separate thoughts. Suddenly there is the shrill ringing of the telephone and Holly jumps to her feet. "That'll be Nick now. He promised to phone."

She lifts the receiver and, although she has been expecting the call, her heart leaps at the sound of his voice.

"Holly darling. How are you? I've been thinking about you all day. I should have stayed with you for the funeral. How did it go? Are you alright?"

"I'm fine. Everything went off well. Sally's staying here to keep me company tonight." She tells him the events of the day. "How are lectures going?"

"Not easy when I'm without you. I miss you so."

"I miss you too."

"I can't wait to see you again. How can I concentrate on wretched anatomy when all I can think of is you?" The words that follow caress her. She thinks how fortunate it is that Sally cannot hear them.

"I'll come down to see you again at the weekend, Holly. Take care. I love you."

"I love you too," she whispers.

When she comes back into the kitchen, Sally notes how her cheeks are flushed with colour and her eyes shining. She can see how Holly's emotions are rocketing from one extreme to the other within minutes.

"Try to keep calm and see what happens, love. Just deal with each day as it comes. I'd better be off to bed now. Mind you don't stay up too long. It's been a long day and you've got an appointment at the bank in the morning, remember."

"I know. The bank manager is going to open Mum's will. He's her executor. Then I'm going to need his help to sort out all my finances as well. I really haven't a clue about anything. Mum dealt with all that after Dad died." Holly sighs apprehensively. "Now I've got to manage everything on my own."

"Well, that's what he's there for, isn't it? Let's wait and see what he's got to say before worrying about it." Sally says goodnight and Holly hears her quick tread as she climbs the stairs to what was Elizabeth's room.

Holly remains sitting motionless at the fireside, lost in thought. She tries not to think of her mother as she is now, buried in the cold dark earth, but recalls the loving, caring woman who brought her up. Despite her frail appearance she always seemed so strong. She was always there whenever Holly came home from school, whenever she had a problem, whenever she needed someone to talk to, but now she has gone and in her place there is an aching void. How will she cope without her mother's strength and support?

Chilled and numb she suddenly awakes with a start. Looking at the clock she realizes that she must have been asleep in the chair for several hours. Her heart feels as lifeless as the dead ashes lying in the grate. When she tries to rise, her legs almost give way beneath her. She stumbles towards the stairs. In her bedroom she goes to stand at the window, staring into the darkness outside, seeing nothing. She has lost her mother and in a sense her father too. She feels as if her very identity has been taken away from her. Whose daughter is she? Where does she belong?

An enormous sadness envelops her like a huge wave. The unshed tears which have been mounting all day break loose and course down her cheeks. She grips the soft silky curtains and buries her face in the familiar pattern of roses. When she raises her eyes at last, the dark sky beyond the hills is already touched with a delicate hue of pale pink. She lies down on the bed, waiting for the day to begin. Perhaps she sleeps again, she does not know.

She cannot say how much later it is when a noise in the kitchen breaks the stillness of the farmhouse. She hears the sound of cinders being raked in the iron grate. Sally is up and bustling about. Soon the fire will be crackling and the kettle on the boil.

A new day has dawned. For her it must be a new beginning. There is no way for her to go except forward. Holly washes quickly in the cold bathroom. There is ice on the window, both inside and out, but when she scratches the pane she can see billowing white clouds sailing like ships across a bright blue sky. When she has dressed, she flings the casement open and takes a deep breath of the wintry air sweeping down from the moors.

She looks at the dale spread out before her, rising up to the moors. Her roots are here. She has never lived anywhere else. The farthest she has ever travelled is to York. This is her world, the world she knows and loves, and yet it is a world which holds no future for her. Suddenly she makes up her mind. Today she is going to speak to the bank manager about selling the farm. Perhaps it will bring enough money for her to be able to study art, perhaps even in London at the Royal College of Art or the Slade. Then she and Nick will be together. She loves him and knows that he loves her. Whatever may come, she feels safe in that knowledge. Perhaps, with his help, she will find out more about the man who was her true father. Who can say what secrets she may uncover?

As she watches, the sun emerges from behind a cloud and floods the dale with golden light. It seems like an omen. She closes the window and goes down to face the new morning.

The town hall clock is striking nine when Holly props her bicycle against the wall of the bank. It is an impressive stone building, and considering the size of the town and the wealth of its inhabitants, disproportionately large. She draws a deep breath, turns the huge brass knob on the door and goes inside. When she has stated the reason for her visit, the clerk at the counter offers her a seat and then returns to the banknotes he is counting, untroubled by both her presence and the absence of customers. While she waits, Holly surveys the wire racks overflowing with brochures. Their content makes her painfully aware that she knows nothing of the state of her financial affairs.

The big hand of the clock on the wall opposite clicks and moves to one minute past nine. As if he has been waiting for its signal, a short dumpy man appears. His portly figure is squeezed into a navy-blue pin-stripe suit with a tie in an incongruously bright shade of red. After they have shaken hands, he shows her into his office.

"Do take a seat, Miss Barton. Please accept my most sincere condolences. I knew your late mother well – such a charming lady." The proprieties having been observed, the bank manager avoids meeting Holly's eyes as he edges between a bulging filing cabinet and a table stacked with thick folders, to his chair. His desk looks surprisingly empty considering the mountains of paperwork that surround it. Only a slim file is lying on the pristine blotting pad. He flicks it open and rifles through its contents while he speaks.

"Here we have all the relevant documents, starting with the will itself." He takes a silver paperknife to slit open a long cream envelope and then removes a sheet of vellum which he unfolds and carefully smoothes out on the desk in front of him. He seems to be relishing the ceremoniousness of the occasion.

"Your late mother had this will drawn up shortly after your father's death. I'll omit the preamble, if I may?" He raises his eyes to glance at her in rhetorical question over the top of his half-moon spectacles, and taking Holly's silence as agreement, he continues. "In her last will and testament Elizabeth Mary Barton, née Fairley, left all her estate, that is the farmhouse, the surrounding out-buildings, the land and all related properties in addition to all her personal possessions to yourself, her only daughter, Holly Barton. A considerable bequest, I may add – at the time." He pauses and looks at the girl sitting in front of him. Her hands are twisting a handkerchief in her lap. His face assumes a softer expression and he lays the will aside.

"Miss Barton," he goes on in a gentler tone of voice, "I do not know how far your mother discussed such matters with you, but the years that followed your father's early death were not easy ones. Most of the land had to be sold off to pay the death duties owing. The remainder, including the house itself, was mortgaged to provide your mother with sufficient means for herself and for your own upbringing and education. Her personal effects are of course untouched by this and there is a small sum in savings certificates, but as your mother did not have any life insurance or other assets, I'm afraid that the house and land, as collateral, must revert to the bank to cover those debts outstanding."

It is easier to use the language of his profession rather than speak plainly to tell this girl in front of him that she has no roof over her head and barely a penny in the world. Holly is sitting with her head bowed. He does not have to look into her eyes. He leans forward and places various forms and documents in front of her while his voice continues to run on monotonously. His soft white hand loosely holds a gold-nibbed fountain pen, which slides over columns of figures, poises over paragraphs, stabs in the air to make a point and finally comes to rest upright in a stand on his desk before he shuffles all the documents together again.

"I'm very sorry, Miss Barton, that I can't give you any more cheering news . . . most distressing . . . no alternative . . . if you have any questions . . . don't hesitate . . . at your service any time." His words wash over Holly like waves. She finds herself outside in the High Street again with no recollection of what she has said or done to get there. When she stares down at the large brown envelope in her hand, it is as if she is seeing it for the first time.

"Oi! Watch out there!" A man carrying a wooden crate full of cauliflowers on one shoulder jostles past her on the pavement. It is market day, though she barely notices the stalls laden with lush green bundles of early vegetables, open boxes of golden daffodils and white narcissi, creamy yellow and orange country cheeses and crates of freshly-caught fish, glittering silver in the morning sunlight. Nor do the cries of the stallholders reach her ears as she pushes her bicycle through bustling crowds of shoppers to the sanctuary of a nearby café. She goes in, orders a cup of coffee and sits down at one of the plastic-topped tables. As she stirs the pale liquid, she tries to collect her thoughts.

She always hoped that she would be able to study art. Even after her mother's death she somehow went on trusting that one day she might be offered a place at one of the art colleges in London, to be near Nick and at the same time study the subject she loves. But now? Now she has to face the fact that she is penniless, or almost so. Her mother's personal things – 'effects' the bank manager called them – are hers. She bites her lip to stop herself from crying at the thought of the little jewellery box containing Elizabeth's engagement ring with its three tiny diamonds, her plain gold watch and a string of pearls which her husband gave her on their first wedding anniversary. She blinks back the tears. The small sum in savings certificates will not last long. She will have to stay on working at the garage; she does not have qualifications for anything else.

Holly raises her cup and sips the unappetising coffee. It is weak and nearly cold. Looking over the rim, she watches a woman come in. Her face has an unhealthy pallor and there is a cigarette hanging from one corner of her mouth. She wheels a crying baby in a pushchair past the table. Holly's eyes follow her, taking in the worn coat, the laddered stockings and the cheap shoes, trodden down at the heel. The child begins to wail and the mother's voice snaps irritably. She can hardly be older than Holly herself, yet her skin is dull, aged beyond her years.

Is that to be her own future? Is that what she might become if she stays in her dead-end job? The realization strikes her like a slap in the face. She stands up so abruptly that she almost knocks her chair over and pushes her way between the tables towards the door. She has to get out. The crowded room is closing in on her. Back in the busy street again she finds herself gasping, drawing deep gulps of fresh air as if to purge her lungs.

She has arranged to meet Flo in the park at eleven and arrives in time to see her friend approaching, her college scarf wrapped round her neck against the cold. She looks so young. Holly feels as if she herself has passed from girlhood to adulthood in the space of only a few days.

Flo sits down on the bench beside her. "Hey!" She turns to face Holly. "You're as white as a sheet. What's the matter? You okay?"

She listens, shocked, as Holly recounts her interview with the bank manager. "And they are even sending someone next week to assess the value of the farm. They want me out of there as soon as I can find somewhere else to go. Oh, Flo!" Her head drops into her hands. "What am I going to do? Where shall I go? I don't earn enough money to rent a place of my own. There's a cousin of my mother's somewhere up in Scotland but I hardly know him, and anyway I don't want to go and live there."

Flo's arm goes round her shoulders. "Come and stay with us. You know my mum and dad would love to have you. We've got masses of space. And it would be great for us to be together."

"It's sweet of you to offer, Flo, but you've got to go back to York. And it's one thing to stay for a couple of days, but I have to find somewhere permanent to live."

"You're coming to our house for supper tonight, aren't you, so let's talk about it then with Mum and Dad. After all," she adds, "it'll only be until you go to art college."

"Art college?" Holly's voice rings with a bitterness that Flo has never heard before. "Art college? I could never afford that! I've hardly a penny to call my own! Maybe I can study at night school or something but there's no way I'm going to get to college now."

For a while neither of them speaks.

"Have you spoken to Nick about all this yet?"

"No, he's at the teaching hospital all day today. He was going to come up on Friday night but there's no point now."

"Now look here," Flo turns to look her friend straight in the eye, "what on earth makes you say that? You told me that he loves you, right?"

Holly nods miserably.

"And he knows you love him too?"

"Yes," Holly admits, thinking that even without teacher-training Flo has already developed the skills she will need to survive in the classroom.

"Well, what does it matter where you live or how much money you've got? If you're really in love, you'll find a way to see each other. Even if you can't be together all the time, you can still love one another!"

Holly stares at her friend. Fancy dear, down-to-earth Flo telling her this! It is she who is normally the romantic one. "I was afraid I might have to give Nick up," she confesses.

"Give him up!" Flo practically snorts. "You might have to give up your home and your wild dreams of studying in London, but there's no reason why you should give up the man you love. Just like there's no reason why you should give me up either!"

For the first time that day Holly smiles.

"I'll phone him tonight . . ."

TWELVE

. . . Holly pulls open the door of the phone box. The stale smell of cold cigarette smoke makes her catch her breath. When she left the Westburys' house on the pretext of wanting to get some fresh air before supper, Flo did not offer to accompany her, understanding that the call Holly is going to make is one that she does not want even her dearest friend to overhear. The phone number of Nick's flat in London is scribbled on a slip of paper in her coat pocket, but she leaves it there. She has looked at it so many times that she knows the figures by heart. She dials. The ringing tone at the other end is faint compared to the pounding of her blood in her head as she presses the receiver to her ear.

An age seems to pass before there is a click, and a man answers. When she asks to speak to Nick Ranleigh, the voice, which must belong to his flatmate, pleasantly offers to go and find him and the sound of footsteps retreating down a hallway follows. From a distance she can hear him calling Nick's name. At last, to her relief, there is his voice in far-off reply, then the sound of him walking towards the phone, picking it up and his polite "Hello?"

"Holly!"

His joy on hearing her is unmistakable. It thrills her whole being, washing comfort over all the pain she has suffered since their separation. One part of her wants to pour out all her worries, another part of her only wants to listen to his voice. She answers his questions briefly. Suddenly the present does not seem to matter; the future will bring them together again. Feeding the phone box with a steady stream of shillings, she tells him about her visit to the bank, all the while expecting his reaction to be as her own has been, yet he remains calm, unaffected.

"When will I see you? When can you come here?" She

knows that she sounds desperate but does not care. The coins are running out now and she has to know when they can meet again before the call is cut off.

He senses her urgency. "As soon as I can get away. I miss you so. Perhaps –" The dialling tone takes over and he is gone.

During supper with the Westburys that evening Holly is quiet and withdrawn. The doctor and his wife warmly repeat Flo's offer that she should live with them and she thanks them, neither accepting nor refusing their invitation. After the meal she cycles back to Black Ridge Farm. The house is cold and empty. It seems too much trouble to light the fire only for herself, so she goes straight to bed.

It is still dark when a sound outside in the yard awakes her. The luminous hands of her alarm clock are pointing to twenty to three. Holly freezes. There is someone outside. A burglar? A prowler? She has never been afraid on the farm at night, but as she suddenly realizes, she has never slept alone here before. There is a further noise, this time a slight scraping sound. Then again. Somebody is at the back door. Her heart is racing. She can hear it thudding in her ears. Can she get to the phone before he gets in? She creeps out of bed, feeling around in the dark for something she can use as a weapon. The poker is in the kitchen grate. Can she get there in time? She hears a click, someone is trying to open the latch on the back door, and then a voice.

"Holly! Are you awake? It's me, Nick!"

She flies down the stairs, nearly falling headlong in her haste, and flings the door open and herself into his arms.

"Wow, this isn't the sort of welcome I expected to get in the middle of the night!" He lifts her off her feet and carries her back inside. "I thought you'd be asleep and get all cross when I woke you up."

"Oh Nick, how could I be? Though I might have killed you because I thought you were a burglar! I've missed you so. I need you so much. But what are you doing here now? I didn't expect you till the weekend. What about all your lectures and tutorials?"

"Damn the lectures and tutorials! When I heard your voice

I just had to come. You sounded so sad. I got in the car as soon as I put the phone down and drove straight here without stopping."

Holly's arms are still round his neck and she nestles her face into the warmth of his coat. As long as they are together, she can face whatever the future may bring.

"I carried you once before, if I remember rightly," he says softly, "and I think I'm getting better with practice. Where do you want me to take you this time?"

"Upstairs, please," she whispers.

A bright sun shining through the bedroom curtains, falling on her face, wakes Holly the next morning. She lies still, not wanting to disturb him as he sleeps in her arms. The kisses and caresses, the words of love and tenderness they have exchanged are like a blanket covering the hurt of the days that have gone before. She looks down at his fair hair lying in unruly curls on his forehead, the sweep of his eyelashes, and his strong hands with their long tapering fingers holding her own. When he finally wakes he opens his grey eyes and smiles at her.

Holly reaches over and switches on the little transistor radio on her bedside table. As usual it is tuned in to one of the off-shore pirate radio stations. The voices of Paul McCartney and John Lennon fill the room . . .

Love, love me do. You know I love you. I'll always be true . . .'

She closes her eyes and he kisses her. "Will you be true, darling?"

"Yes, I will," she whispers, and his lips descend on hers once again.

An hour later, after Nick has managed to light the fire in the kitchen range, they are drinking coffee in bed. "Let's go out in the car. It's a fantastic day so we can have the hood down," Nick suggests. "Leave all your worries behind you. Doctor's orders!"

Holly throws back the covers at once. The prospect of escaping from her present situation, if only for a short while, is almost as good as the thought of spending the day with Nick.

"Where are we going?" she asks, as the car bumps over the ruts in the lane that leads into the town.

"Wherever you want. To the end of the world if you like."

To the end of the world! If only he could take her there. Despite her worries she feels an irrational sense of well-being. As long as she has Nick, everything will be alright. "Let's go to Sands End again."

In answer he swerves the car to the left at the Market Cross and soon they are speeding over the moors towards the coast. It is a glorious spring day with a brisk breeze that sends clouds flying like white balloons across a sky of the brightest blue. Moorland sheep raise their heads briefly as they pass, chewing contently, then lower them again to resume their search for early shoots of fresh grass among the heather.

At the top of Lythe Bank, the vast sweep of the bay at Sands End appears before them. They park at the bottom of the hill again but this time the tide is in so they walk hand in hand along the sea front, stopping now and then to lean on the railings and gaze out over the water. Huge waves roll up to the sea-wall, only to break and be sucked back into the green depths before rolling in again, a never-ending cycle of movement that makes Holly feel small and insignificant. She pauses, staring at the horizon, hoping that Nick will not notice that her eyes have filled with tears.

What is the matter? Why is she so blissfully happy one moment and desperately sad the next? She seems to be at the mercy of her emotions. She feels like a tiny boat tossing far out on an angry sea, or a plane flying out of control with no land in sight.

Suddenly there are drops of rain, at first as fine as spray from the waves, but then they see that a single grey cloud has pushed its way in front of the sun. The spots are coming more quickly now, faster and faster, blurring their vision as they run towards the car. Inside they sit listening as they splatter on the canvas hood. The day which began so fine seems to be taking a different turn in every sense.

Nick notes Holly's change of mood. "We look like two pensioners on a day out," he jokes, pouring coffee from the flask they have brought and handing her a plastic cup. She takes it gratefully, wrapping her hands around it for warmth, and smiles at his attempt to cheer her up, wanting him to think he has succeeded. He opens a paper bag of rolls they stopped to buy at a bakery on the way, and offers it to her, but she shakes her head. He takes one himself and bites into it hungrily. They sit in silence, a comfortable silence as if they have known each other for years instead of weeks. When they have finished their coffee, Nick turns the key in the engine and looks at her inquiringly. "And now?"

"Let's go to Rosedale. It's so lovely there. I haven't been since . . ." She hesitates. "It was one of the last trips Dad took Mum and me on . . . just before he died," she adds so softly that he barely hears her words.

As a child she always looked forward to Sunday afternoons, the one time in the week when neither of her parents had to work. Her mother used to put on her hat and best suit – her 'costume' she called it, her father would get the battered Ford Popular out of the barn and they would all set off to explore one of the dales. They would take a picnic and eat it in some woodland glade beside a stream, except in winter when they sat in the car. Afterwards, while her mother relaxed, Holly and her father played French cricket, walked in the woods or searched for minnows, sticklebacks, newts and tadpoles in hidden brooks and pools. She can still feel the sharp bite of the water, crystal-clear and ice-cold running over her toes, still smell the heady scent of may blossom, heavy like snow on the hawthorn boughs, still see the bluebells rippling like a river in the breeze, and still taste the soft vanilla ice-cream that they used to buy on their way home when the day was drawing to its close. Then there would be Sunday tea, always with something special – a cake, meringues or jelly – but somehow the meal never tasted as good as it should, because it marked the fact that Sunday with all its joys was over and school would have to be faced in the morning.

The time passes quickly. Lost in her thoughts and memories, Holly can later only dimly recall the winding lanes they follow, dipping into the valleys of rolling dales where pretty cottages around village greens lie sheltered from the storms that buffet the moors. In Farndale they stop at a pub where Nick insists on ordering a bowl of soup for her, and though she is not hungry she eats it to please him. When they come outside again, the rain has stopped and a watery sun has appeared, so they take a walk to see the wild daffodils, but the winter has been too cold and, disappointingly, few have opened their golden heads.

When they draw up outside Black Ridge Farm it is late afternoon. Nick stops the car and switches off the engine. The sudden silence jolts Holly out of her reverie. "I'm sorry, I haven't been much fun today." She gives him a weak smile.

"Holly." Nick leans forward with both arms on the steering wheel, turning his head to face her. The grey eyes meet her own. "Do you really think I expect you to be fun all the time? Your mum's died, you've had that news about your father and you're about to lose your home! Of course you're sad and worried. If I've helped you relax just a bit today, then I'm happy." He kisses the end of her nose. "You okay now?"

"Okay," she whispers.

"Is it alright if I go now? I've got a tutorial I can't miss in the morning."

"Of course. Thanks so much for coming."

He takes her in his arms and she feels all the warmth and passion of his kiss. "I'll be back again as soon as I can. Phone me tomorrow night. Promise?"

"I promise."

She gets out and slams the door. With a roar of the engine the car disappears round the bend in the lane, leaving her alone. Slowly she turns and enters the house. The kitchen is as they left it, their coffee mugs of the morning bearing silent witness to his visit. Holly puts them in the sink and turns on the tap to fill the kettle. No sooner does the water begin to flow than something snaps within her brain and she turns it off again.

She cannot go on like this, waiting for something to happen, waiting for other people – the Westburys, the bank manager, Nick, whoever – to take charge of her life. She has to do something herself. She has to make her own decisions. She has to start taking control. Spinning on her heel, she grabs her coat and pulls it on, closing the kitchen door behind her as she goes out. She does not stop to lock it but turns towards the moors. She runs, walks, stumbles and climbs until, panting and almost exhausted, she reaches the crags where she met Nick for the first time. She did not know when she set off that she would be coming here, but when she throws herself onto the dry heather under the rocks, she knows why she has come.

All day Nick wanted to take her away from her grief and problems, yet every place they visited had the opposite effect, drawing her back into the life she has led so far, reviving memories of times gone by and people she has lost. Up here she is free at last, free to breathe, free to look ahead, free to decide her future.

Yet it is crazy to be up here, she tells herself. The wind has dropped for the first time that day, the clouds have disappeared and the sun is setting, bathing the moors with golden rays, but the light is fading rapidly. She will have to find her way back in the dark. It will not be easy but she knows she will manage. A strength and confidence fill her which she has not felt since her mother died. It is as if, during all the day with Nick, her thoughts have been unconsciously moving in one particular direction, like a strong undercurrent pulsing through a river that seems quite smooth and placid. Now those thoughts are bursting through like bubbles to the surface of her mind.

She makes herself consider her alternatives rationally. She can keep her job at the garage, stay with the Westburys until she has found a small flat of her own that she can afford to rent – and then? What future would that be?

What if – she hardly dares voice her thoughts even to herself – what if she should leave all this behind her? With 'all this' her eyes take in the moors, the dales and all her former life spread out before her. What if she follows the idea which has been forming in her brain ever since her mother died?

Perhaps she can study art in London after all.

She summons up all the arguments she can think of against her plan. She has not got the qualifications to apply for a place at college. Perhaps she has not got enough talent either and she certainly has not got enough money. She is virtually penniless and on her own with no one to help her.

Yet even as these thoughts enter her head, she refutes them. She knows she can make it. She will take a preparatory course, at night school perhaps, to learn more, develop, get a portfolio of work together so that she can apply to one of the London art schools. And as for money, when she gets a place at college she can apply for a grant, and if that is not enough she can take a job. Any job will be better than what she is doing now. And she is not alone in the world. She has Nick. In London they can be together, she can share in his life and he in hers.

And one day, when she has reached her goal, she will go to Paris and trace Philippe. She knows she will always love Tom Barton but she has to know more about her real father, the man her mother loved so deeply. She is Philippe's daughter, she is half-French. Is that why the language comes to her so easily? In finding out more about him, she will learn more about herself. Despite her love for the moors and dales she has always felt that somehow she does not quite belong, that her future lies elsewhere. This is her chance to find out.

Holly gets to her feet. She is perfectly calm, her decision made. She has everything to gain and nothing to lose. The rays of the setting sun are casting long shadows at her feet. It is already too dark to go down the way she climbed up. She hopes she can remember where Nick led her on the day they met. She takes her first step forward, not knowing where the path will lead . . .

THIRTEEN

Paris, Spring 1967

The rue du Vieux Moulin had seen better days. Holly walked down the avenue of once-stately villas with peeling paintwork and battered shutters until she reached number 22. She opened the rusty iron gate and went up a narrow pathway overgrown with weeds. A night of steady rainfall had given the house an air of sadness. Dripping bushes on either side leaned inwards to touch her, showering her with cold drops of water as she passed. A thorny tangle of unpruned roses arched over the porch as if to catch the unsuspecting visitor unawares. This solidly-built house had once been the home of a worthy bourgeois family with a cook and a butler, parlour maids and kitchen maids, perhaps a nursemaid for the children, but now a tattered array of name-plates in various colours and handwriting told a different story.

Holly found the name she was seeking. Faded letters on a white card said simply *Valmont*. There was no title, no first name, no 'de' to show its owner's standing. Weak with nervousness she pushed the button next to it and heard a bell ring. Monsieur de Valmont lived on the ground floor, it seemed. There was no reply from within. Her heart sank. She rang again. Finally she heard the sound of feet shuffling towards the door.

"J'arrive," a quavering male voice announced. A bolt was drawn back, the door opened slowly and she found herself face to face with an elderly man. Despite his age his silvery hair was thick, and he did not stoop but stood tall and upright, staring straight at her.

Holly had prepared a little speech of introduction but found herself unable to say a word. The old gentleman was equally silent. His watery eyes did not leave her face.

"Geneviève," he stammered. "Geneviève, c'est toi." He seemed to have mistaken her for someone else. He had turned pale. Holly was afraid he might be about to faint or have a heart attack. She decided she had better clear up the situation as quickly as possible.

She introduced herself. "Excuse me, monsieur. I'm trying to find out some information about the Valmont family. May I come in and ask you a few questions? It won't take long."

He did not answer but stepped aside to allow her to enter and showed her down a long passageway into a small sitting-room where a radio was playing. He turned it off and they faced each other in silence again. Without being asked, Holly sat down on a worn sofa, noting that it was antique. She cast her eyes around. All the furniture was Louis Seize, but all of it was in an equally dilapidated state. There was no fire in the grate and, though the room was spotlessly clean, it was chill and damp. Guy de Valmont sat down opposite her. He could not have expected her visit but he was impeccably dressed. Yet his clothes – a tweed jacket, cavalry twill trousers, Oxford shirt and striped tie – had the same air of impoverished gentility as his home.

"What can I do for you, mademoiselle?" His voice was stronger now but his eyes had still not left her face. Holly began to feel awkward. What if she had come all this way and intruded on this stranger's privacy for nothing? She decided to be brief. "When I lived in England, monsieur, I was given this." She handed him the drawing of her mother, signed 'P. de V.'.

Guy de Valmont stared intently at the sketch. "Who gave you this?"

"It belonged to my mother. When she died, it was given to me."

"Elizabeth is dead?" He raised his eyes to meet her own and Holly saw them fill with tears. Her heart stood still.

"You knew my mother?" she managed to whisper.

The old gentleman shook his head sadly. "We never met her. It was Geneviève's greatest wish to get to know her. Our son, Philippe, had told us so much about Elizabeth in his letters, but after he was killed there was no way we could get in touch. We never found out what happened to her."

"Geneviève was your wife?"

Guy de Valmont nodded, pulled a handkerchief out of the pocket of his jacket and wiped his eyes.

"And, Monsieur, you are absolutely sure that your son had a relationship with my mother, Elizabeth Fairley?"

"Yes. Philippe had been fighting with the Free French during the war and in 1943 he was working for de Gaulle in London. It was while he was there that he met this lovely girl, Elizabeth, one evening at the Café de Paris. He wrote and told us all about her. Geneviève and I were delighted. We so much wanted him to be happy. He was our only son." Tears began to run down his thin cheeks.

"What happened?" Holly wanted to hear more although she could hardly bear to listen.

"He was killed on March the fifteenth in London in 1944. He was on official business for de Gaulle and the motorcycle he was riding skidded off the wet road and hit a lamp post. There was no one else involved, no one to blame. It was just one of those terrible, meaningless things that happen. Geneviève never recovered from the shock. She had always been frail. She died within a year."

Holly rose and went towards him. She gently laid an arm round his shaking shoulders till gradually his sobs subsided.

"You know who I am, don't you?"

"I knew the minute I saw you on the doorstep," he said. "You are Philippe and Elizabeth's daughter." He stood up. "Come with me. I have something to show you."

He led her by the hand into the next room. It was furnished just as sparsely as the sitting-room, bare except for a chest of drawers and a single bed, but on the wall between two long windows that gave onto the garden, there was a large oil painting. It was a full-length, life-size portrait of a woman in evening dress.

Holly stared at the painting and gasped. She seemed to be

looking at a slightly older version of herself, as she might perhaps look in ten years' time.

The woman's hair was dark brown like her own, but cut to a chin-length bob falling in elaborate waves that were caught at one side in a diamond clasp. She was the same height as herself and slender, wearing an elegant gown of lilac silk in the fashion of the thirties, which clung to her perfect figure. A stole of silver fox fur fell gracefully from one of her shoulders. Her head was turned towards the artist, who had caught the slight smile playing on her red lips and the sparkle in her clear, brown eyes. She wore no other jewellery, but her slim hands held a single crimson rose.

Guy de Valmont was looking at the painting with love in his eyes. "Geneviève!" he said softly.

"My grandmother!" Holly's emotions overwhelmed her. She was unable to speak.

Guy de Valmont took her hand once more and led her towards a small table that stood beside the bed. He picked up a photograph in a sliver frame and gave it to her. "Philippe," he said quietly.

She saw the same handsome man in his mid-twenties who was in the portrait her mother had treasured, but this time he was in military uniform. She was still holding the photograph when they returned to the sitting-room. Guy de Valmont offered her a chair at a dining table on which he placed two delicate, intricately-cut wine glasses, and disappeared. When he returned he was bearing a dusty bottle wreathed with cobwebs.

"Château de Valmont," he said proudly. "The last bottle from the grapes of our vineyards. I have been keeping it for an occasion such as this." He uncorked it, sniffed the cork appreciatively and poured out the rich, golden liquid. "Ma chère petite-fille." He raised his glass to hers. "Let us drink to our family, the Valmonts, and to you, my dear, who have brought me such joy. If only your dear grand-mère could have lived to be here with us today."

The cool liquid slipped down her throat. The vintage wine

was as bitter-sweet as their meeting. Guy de Valmont reached inside his jacket pocket and took out a worn leather wallet. He fingered inside and withdrew a letter. He must have read it countless times, the paper was so brittle and thin. When he unfolded it, it was cracked at the fold. He handed it to her. "This was the last letter our son sent us before he was killed."

It was written in French, with long, sloping characters, so faded that she could barely decipher what they said. Her father wrote joyfully of Elizabeth, the lovely English girl he had met, of her beauty and the sweetness of her nature, of his plans to bring her home to France and marry her. At the close of the letter he told his parents of their engagement and asked for their blessing. Tears were streaming down Holly's face when she came to the closing expressions of love which Philippe sent to his mother and father from himself and his fiancée.

Three hours passed, at times sadly when her grandfather told her about the fortunes of the Valmont family, at times gaily when he told her about her father's mischievous character and some of the pranks he had played as a child. She tried to explain the meaning of her name and he could not understand why anyone should be called after what he called "a prickly plant". At last he became serious. "I am sorry, je suis désolé, my dear granddaughter, that I have no fortune to give to you, nothing of value to leave to you. Our family's château, our land and our vineyards have all been sold."

Holly was horrified. "Please, grand-père, don't think I've come looking for you to gain something. You mustn't think that! I don't want you to give me anything! You have already given me so much." He looked puzzled. "You have given me my identity. At last I know who I really am. That means more to me than any inheritance."

"The name de Valmont is an inheritance in itself," he replied. "Will you accept it, my dear? Perhaps you will marry one day, but until you do, will you bear the name of our family?"

"Give me a little time, grandfather," she begged. "That's not something I can decide now." She thought of Tom and

Elizabeth Barton and how much she owed to them. She did not believe that she could give up their name so easily. "I'll think about it," she promised. He seemed to understand although she did not explain.

Their long talk and the emotions of the afternoon had tired him immensely. He clutched her arm for support as she rose to leave. "Come back to see me soon, my dear."

Holly kissed him on both cheeks. "Of course I will."

When the door had closed behind her, she realized that she too was exhausted. Slowly she made her way towards the Métro, found her way to the platform and sat down on a bench. All of a sudden she felt numb, almost in shock, and strangely unable to register any particular feeling.

The close affinity that she had always felt towards this country, its people, its culture and its language now made sense. Everything was falling into place. Part of her roots were here. She was the last member of a great and noble family. She thought with tenderness of her grandfather; there was already a rapport between them which would deepen in time.

She was no longer alone. The realization had not come like a sudden flash but diffused gradually like a warm glow through her body. She did not know how long she sat there, but when she rose at last her heart was filled with happiness.

Alone in her tiny room that evening, she pushed open the shutters and leant out of the window, gazing at the lights of the city. The illuminated Sacré-Cœur basilica stood like a white ghost on the hill of Montmartre, the colourful neon signs of Pigalle below in garish contrast to its cool beauty. A soft breath of air touched her skin and the murmur of the city rose towards her. Even at this hour the boulevards with their cafés and restaurants were alive. Soon home-going revellers would meet incoming office workers and the air would be filled with the smell of baking bread and the sound of gushing torrents of water sluicing the streets, a cycle of life forever perpetuating itself.

She was resting her flushed cheek against the window frame when a tap on the door broke into her thoughts.

"Entrez."

It was Marie. "Excusez-moi, mademoiselle. Madame is calling you on the phone in the salon."

Holly rushed down to the floor below. She had quite forgotten that Arlette had promised to ring her. She pressed the receiver closer to one ear, blocking the other with her finger, all her efforts concentrated on making out the words coming over the crackling line. The French telephone service was never particularly reliable and the connection to Milan was atrocious that evening.

"Holly, can you hear me?" At the other end Arlette had abandoned her ladylike manner and was shouting at the top of her voice to make herself understood. "I've heard that the photos for the knitwear feature have turned out wonderfully. Congratulations, my dear! You did really well."

"Thank you, Arlette, but it's Jean-Pierre and the girls who should get the credit. They were brilliant. When do you expect to be back here?"

"Not until Saturday. There's a textile manufacturer I have to visit before I leave. The fabrics here – oh my dear! I wish you could have been with me, they are so gorgeous – the designs, the colours, the . . ." A loud buzzing interrupted her rapturous ramblings. "So please can you – "

Arlette's voice could be heard issuing rapid instructions regarding the article for the magazine feature she wished Holly to write on her behalf. Then the line crackled again and, just when Holly expected it to break down completely, Arlette's voice unexpectedly surged through once more.

". . . know you'll enjoy the dinner on Friday evening. It's so much more appropriate for you to go. It would be such a pity otherwise and Julien will be so disa. . ."

Julien's feelings remained undescribed because a babble of Italian voices crowded in on the line. After waiting in vain for several minutes, Holly reluctantly put down the phone.

She had heard sufficient to understand what Arlette meant. The merchant bank of which Julien was a junior executive was going to celebrate its bi-centenary, an event which was to be crowned with a private dinner at the famous Lapérousse restaurant. He had invited Arlette to the event to recompense her for the many evenings he had spent at her home, but she had graciously insisted that he should be seen in such circles with a younger guest, someone nearer his own age. Surely Holly would be the ideal partner for him? Holly's protests had gone unheeded at the time and she even secretly wondered whether Arlette's prolonged sojourn in Milan was a way of ensuring that she should take her place at the dinner.

Until now she had not been particularly keen on the prospect of spending an evening with Julien's banking colleagues and their wives, but the more she thought about it, the more she began to look forward to what would surely be a glamorous event. Arlette had ensured that her appearance would be flawless and her French was good enough now for her to contemplate the formal occasion among strangers with even a thrill of anticipation. The happenings of the day bathed everyone and everything around her in a rosy glow.

No sooner had she put the phone down than it rang again. This time it was Julien, charming as ever, expressing his delight that she was to be his date. He had not visited her once during Arlette's absence, but Holly knew that his appearance at the apartment when she was known to be alone, without Arlette acting as chaperone, would have provoked a scandal among the elderly neighbours and greatly shocked the concierge. It would also have damaged Arlette's own reputation, which, as a widow living alone, she was at pains to preserve. Holly had lived in France long enough to know that its people, despite their reputation for love and romance, were deeply prudish, if not to say Victorian, in their attitudes. He announced that he would pick her up in a taxi at eight o'clock on Friday evening, and rang off.

Holly was relieved that Arlette had been so far-seeing as to arrange what she was to wear on such a grand occasion. Her own wardrobe contained nothing that would have been in the least suitable, but she knew that the deep-red chiffon gown hanging in her bedroom would give her confidence even had it not borne a Dior label, and Marie had promised to put her hair up for her.

The rest of the week passed quickly as Holly worked on the feature for the magazine. She wanted the article with the photos and the captions to be perfect. The deadline was Friday, and when she finally submitted her work she was sure that Arlette would be satisfied with the result. Relieved that it was done, she thought she deserved a celebration and excitedly contemplated the evening to come.

FOURTEEN

At eight that evening, Holly stood in front of the mirror in her room, staring at her reflection. A graceful, self-confident young woman in a gown of red chiffon spangled with silver met her gaze. Where was the English girl who had arrived in Paris so frightened and insecure two years ago? Had she really changed as much as her outward appearance suggested? One day she would have to leave this dress and all the luxury it embodied behind, and then she would find out. She wondered when that day would be, before dismissing the thought from her head with a toss of the loose curls that cascaded from the silver clasp in her dark hair. She was not going to think about her future now. She just wanted to enjoy herself tonight.

As she reached for her silver clutch bag and her wrap, there was a tap on the door. For a moment she thought it might be Julien and was most amused to find herself quite shocked at the idea. It was Marie who entered the room.

"Monsieur de Mervais has arrived and is waiting in the salon, mademoiselle. Je vous souhaite une bonne soirée."

Holly ran lightly down the stairs to the floor below to greet him. As she passed the table in the hallway, her eye fell on a pale blue airmail envelope lying there. The large round characters on it were unmistakable: a letter from Flo! The temptation to go back to her room and read it almost got the better of her but she did not want to keep Julien waiting. She slipped it unopened into her evening bag.

When she entered the salon Julien's eyes shone with admiration and he abandoned his fluent English in favour of his native tongue. "Bonsoir, Holly. Mais tu es ravissante!" He emphasized the compliment by raising her outstretched hand to his lips.

"Bonsoir, Julien." Holly's brown eyes danced. She could see

that Julien was going to subject her to the full power of his charm tonight. She decided that she would take up the challenge. What better way to enjoy herself in this city of romance than flirting with a handsome young aristocrat?

The evening in the noble restaurant began as she had expected. A champagne reception during which several lengthy speeches were made was followed by a lavish meal. Holly was seated on Julien's right at a round table with three other junior executives and their wives or girlfriends. In accompaniment to the succession of excellent dishes of rich French cuisine, the wines flowed freely and soon the laughter from their table was making heads turn in their direction. Julien and his colleagues all agreed that the event was unbearably stuffy and made plans to escape at the first opportunity. Holly thought that this might not make a good impression on his superiors but did not feel bound to say so if he did not recognize this himself. In fact, she was coming to realize that Julien had a pronounced tendency to use his family's name and wealth as a ticket to behaving more or less as he wanted. When he told her they were leaving for somewhere more exciting, she rose to her feet with the others and, although coffee, cigars and liqueurs had only just been served, amid disapproving frowns from the neighbouring tables their party left the room.

Their taxi sped along the Champs-Elysées, then made its way through the elegant eighth arrondissement before stopping in front of a long striped awning that led to a pair of glass doors. A uniformed commissionaire leapt to open them at their approach, and Julien's hand at her elbow guided Holly up a flight of red-carpeted stairs to where, he assured her, they would find the newest, hottest night-spot in Paris.

Inside, she caught her breath in surprise. She had the overwhelming impression of being spirited away to a desert island. Palm tree fronds waved gently over brightly-decorated tables. A profusion of exotic blooms filled the warm air with a sweet, heavy scent, and stars winked softly overhead in the velvety sky of a tropical night. A West Indian combo playing lilting Caribbean rhythms lulled her senses.

Régine, the club owner and uncrowned queen of Parisian nightlife, approached them smiling. "Julien, how wonderful to see you." Standing on tiptoe she raised her lips to kiss him swiftly on both cheeks before she turned to face Holly. Despite the warmth of the welcome, Holly distinctly felt herself to be of only minor interest in her role as Julien's latest conquest. He seemed to be acquainted with a great many of the other guests and Holly felt both appraising and appreciative glances from members of the jeunesse dorée as he led her to their table that directly adjoined the dance floor.

"Do you come here often?" Holly hoped that the only question which came into her mind did not sound as banal in French as it did in English.

"Sometimes," Julien said vaguely, his eyes scanning the couples on the dance floor. Then he seemed to remember his manners and turned towards her, his lips widening in a brilliant smile. "But never in company as lovely as this."

It was a game they were playing, Holly realized, a superficial game in which flattery and words meant more than truth and feelings, a game played for romance, not for love. Well, she was prepared to play his game, just for tonight. She simply wanted to have a good time and make the most of the whole beguiling experience. Moving in his arms to the insinuating rhythms, she relaxed. Julien was at his most delightful and his seeming ignorance of the fact that on all sides beautiful exquisitely-dressed girls were trying to catch his eye, flattered her. He drew her closer, whispering compliments as they danced.

The music stopped, and as a group of limbo dancers took the floor, Julien led her to the bar, a beach hut lavishly festooned with orchids. Gaily refusing all the barman's efforts to ply her with fruit-laden cocktails of rainbow hue, Holly accepted a glass of champagne. She raised her glass.

"A nous – to us," Julien breathed, his black eyes glinting over the sparkling liquid.

Suddenly he spun round as a heavy hand descended on his shoulder. "Julien, mon vieux. What are you doing here? I thought you'd be at that ghastly do your company's running tonight. And who's this lovely lady? Won't you introduce me?"

"Olivier, hi. We came on here after the dinner." Julien's voice barely concealed his annoyance at this interruption. "Holly, this is Olivier Pascal. We were at university together. Olivier, this is Holly Barton."

"American?" he inquired abruptly.

"No, I'm from England."

"Ah, Anglaise." Olivier's tone had dropped in an insolent manner that showed his distinct lack of interest. He turned his attention back to Julien, blatantly disregarding her presence. "I was trying to get through to you all afternoon, my friend, but you weren't at your desk. The latest figures from the Bourse all point to a . . ."

She could see that Julien was acutely embarrassed by this crass rudeness towards her, but oblivious of having committed any faux-pas, Olivier had now taken his arm and was immersed in a recital of the latest stock market developments. Since Julien found no way of extracting himself from Olivier's limpet-like grip or cutting short his soliloquy, Holly thought she had better come to his aid.

"Excuse me, Julien. I'll be back in a minute."

Olivier barely acknowledged her departure, but Julien thanked her wordlessly with a look which said that he would free himself of this tiresome intruder at the first opportunity.

In the restroom Holly decided to check her hair and makeup, knowing that she would have to wait a while until Julien was alone again. When she opened her bag a thrill of pleasure went through her at the sight of Flo's letter. She sat down on the velvet stool in front of the vanity to enjoy it.

Flo began by describing Sally's funeral – how many people had attended and how wonderfully the vicar had spoken of all the help and devotion the little nurse had given to the community. Soon she moved on to happier themes and Holly's lips curled into a smile as she read Flo's cheerful tales of the ups and downs she was going through during her teaching practice.

Every word showed Holly that her friend would bring the same energy and dedication to her profession as Sally had done. Then Flo wrote of Mike's work on the farm, and Holly could almost feel the cool, fresh wind from the moors blowing across the green fields in the dale with their early shoots of wheat.

The sensation was so real that, when she had finished reading, she remained sitting very still. Slowly she raised her eyes from the letter to the mirror and was shocked to see a stranger there. A full second passed before she realized that she was looking at herself. She was this woman in the red dress that did not belong to her, on a date with a man who meant nothing to her. She stared at her reflection. Was that her? What was she doing here? Who in truth was she? What did she really want? She could not say.

In a sudden flash of awareness she saw that all her life she had been playing a role – just as she was playing a role tonight. A succession of roles played to please other people: the dutiful daughter and diligent schoolgirl, the admiring girlfriend and understanding partner, the helpful assistant and gracious guest. She had always been 'charming and courteous', three words in one of her school reports that had made her mother prouder than if she had gained top marks in all subjects. Perhaps it was time to stop simply wanting to be liked? Perhaps it was time to find out who she, Holly Barton, really was and what she wanted from her life? Before it was too late.

She suddenly realized how long she had been sitting, deep in thought. Julien must be wondering where she was. Quickly she made her way back to their table.

"Holly! I was beginning to think that you'd deserted me!" Julien rose to greet her on her return. "Mais tu es pâle, you've gone quite pale. Are you well?"

"Only rather tired. It's been a long day."

"Have a little more champagne to revive you. When I see Arlette again, I'll tell her that she's making you work too hard," he said with mock severity as he poured the sparkling liquid into her glass.

Holly watched the bubbles forming like seed pearls. "Be careful," she thought, "you're playing his game again. Stop while you can."

She felt the prickling wine touch her lips and flow down her throat. Then the thoughts which had been in her head only minutes before began to burst like the bubbles in her glass. Why could she not think clearly? Maybe she really was too tired. Maybe she had drunk too much wine. She could not make any decisions now. She would think about all that in the morning. This evening she just wanted to enjoy herself.

Was it one, two or three hours later? Holly could not say. She was barely aware of the taxi speeding through the emptiness of the boulevards in the cold grey light of early morning. Julien's arm was around her, her head lay heavily on his shoulder, and her hair had come loose and spread over the soft cashmere of his coat. Murmured words and the rustle of a note as he paid the cab driver roused her from a half-sleep. She was dimly conscious of the fact that their journey had ended not at Arlette's home on the Ile Saint-Louis but in front of a tall apartment block.

Standing unsteadily on the pavement in the cold night air, she realized that she did not know where she was. What was happening? She clung to Julien's arm as he led her inside the building. His other hand fumbled in the inner pocket of his coat to produce a key which he inserted into a slot by the elevator. Within seconds they were whisked smoothly and noiselessly up to the top floor. He opened the door to his penthouse, led Holly inside and took her wrap. She felt dizzy and weird, almost as if she were watching herself from some distant place, somewhere outside her own body. As she crossed to sit down on a couch beside the window, the floor seemed to be swaying.

She looked around her. The spacious room was furnished with a minimum of ultra-modern pieces in white and chrome. The effect was cool, elegant and very expensive, but it was the huge panoramic window that caught her attention. She gazed out at the magnificent view. Julien came and stood behind her. A full minute passed before either of them spoke.

"How beautiful!"

She thought she had seen all aspects of this lovely city, yet she was unprepared for the breathtaking vision that lay at her feet. Like a sleeping giant, Paris stretched out before her. The silver serpent of the Seine wound its way through its heart. The tree-lined Champs-Elysées could be seen leading to the great Étoile with the illuminated Arc de Triomphe, from where the elegant boulevards radiated in all directions. Holly recalled a French teacher long ago telling the class that these broad straight avenues had been conceived to allow cavalry charges to quell street riots and control the political uprisings of a seething nineteenth-century populace. How strange that she should remember that now. Despite its beauty, the city seemed to take on a sinister aspect.

Soft music broke in on her thoughts and Julien was kissing the back of her neck. "Welcome to my world," he whispered, and as she turned to face him he took her into his arms, pulling her closer. He was moving sensuously against her in a way that was totally different from how they had previously danced. His hands were caressing her body through the thin chiffon of her dress, moving down her back towards her buttocks, pressing her to him. Then his fingers found the zip of her gown and Holly felt the light fabric fall away from her shoulders and sink softly to the floor. Standing in her silk camisole and stockings, she was lifted off her feet and carried effortlessly to the bed in an adjoining room. She had no power to resist.

The dark eyes seemed to hypnotise her, black pools in which she was drowning as he bent over her. He whispered words no man had said to her before, words that shocked her even as they made her senses spin. Thought became impossible as his lips covered her own, his tongue flickering into her mouth, exploring, becoming more and more insistent. His hands, slowly at first, then hurriedly, began to pull eagerly at the lace straps of her dessous, ripping the delicate silk and exposing her breasts. His head descended and his teeth bit into her flesh, his hands roughly forcing her shoulders back onto the pillows.

Danger lights flashed in her brain. Something had gone desperately, horribly wrong. It should not be like this; this was not what she wanted. Julien was half undressed, one hand loosening the rest of his clothing, the other arm pinning her down, heaving himself on to her body.

"No," she pleaded. "No, Julien. No! Stop! Don't! You're hurting me."

Her voice only seemed to rouse his passion further. His hands now held her wrists tightly above her head, his burning eyes fixed on her naked body as she twisted and struggled to free herself.

"Non, ma petite Holly. I will show you how we make love here. A little excitement, non? You are a woman. You are too old for high school petting now."

"Julien, let me go! Please! Not like this. No!"

She was no match for him. His powerful knee thrust her legs apart. The weight of his chest crushed her own. She screamed when he entered her, almost passing out with shock and pain, but her cries only seemed to heighten his arousal. His body was pounding against hers, his breath coming in gasps that rasped in her ear, his grip holding her so tightly she felt her wrists would snap. With a spasmodic lurch, he was still, his energy spent. He rolled from her onto his back and lay motionless, staring at the ceiling.

"And that, ma petite Anglaise, was a little lesson. Do not flirt with a Frenchman if you do not wish to start a fire."

He turned towards her. She could not move. She felt violated and besmirched. Slowly her eyes filled with tears and she was amazed to see his face soften. "Perhaps it was a little hard, my French lesson today. It will not hurt so much next time, ma petite. I confess I was carried away by your beauty. I promise to be more of a gentleman when we make love again."

"Again?" Holly's paralysis vanished. She rounded on him incredulously. "You call that love? Are you mad? Do you really imagine that I'd let you anywhere near me again?" Somehow she found the strength to scramble from the bed, pulling her torn garments together, struggling into her evening gown.

He lay propped up on one elbow watching her in idle amusement. "Of course you will, chérie. You'll be back for more before long."

Holly did not attempt to reply. She was terrified that he might prevent her from leaving, that he might attack her again. But he made no move to stop her from going. She grabbed her wrap and bag, flung open the door of the apartment and slammed it behind her. As she ran towards the elevator she seemed to hear the hollow echo of mocking laughter.

A vacant taxi was passing and she managed to flag it down. She gave the driver the address of Arlette's apartment, realizing that she had absolutely no idea which part of the city she was in. As she sat in the back, the driver sped through unfamiliar, deserted streets. Holly closed her eyes. She was trembling from head to toe. She pulled her wrap more tightly round her body but even the stuffy warmth inside the car could not take away the icy chill that gripped her. The driver kept glancing at her through his rear-view mirror, clearly wondering whether she was ill or drunk. He tried to start a conversation. Perhaps he wanted to help her, but she simply ignored him. Her body ached, but the physical pain was nothing compared to the mental torture. How could Julien, who had always behaved like the perfect gentleman, have treated her like this? What had come over him? How could he stoop so low? How could an evening that started out so well lead to such a horrific ending? What had turned him into such a monster that he could do this to her? The questions tumbled over one another inside her head, but even as they did so, other questions started to surface.

Had he always been so perfect? Holly remembered how he had kissed her the evening after their visit to the Comédie Française. There had been something violent about him then, something which had frightened her and made her draw away. During the whole of their relationship he had sought to dominate her, down to the tiniest details. And what about Arlette's warning? Had Arlette not tried to tell her about his true character? Had she taken her words seriously enough? And what about all the other signs? The way those women in the night club had looked at him. How many of them had had affairs with him? And that man, Olivier – looking back, his attitude towards her seemed to show that he knew how Julien treated his women.

What about Julien himself? The very thought of him revolted her, but suddenly, for the first time, she saw him as he really was. Anyone in his position – good-looking, rich and single – would not be without a partner unless there was something seriously wrong, unless that person was incapable of forming a genuine relationship, unless that person was so sick that he could only find pleasure in inflicting pain. He was perverted, she saw now, but she had been too stupid, too naïve to notice.

There was a wet, sticky feeling between her legs. Perhaps she was bleeding. Perhaps she should tell the taxi driver to take her to a hospital so that she could prove that she had been raped, and take legal action against him. The idea was tempting, but she quickly dropped it. The scandal it would cause would inevitably involve Arlette and she had already made up her mind that Arlette must never know what had happened. Holly knew that the kind-hearted Frenchwoman had become very fond of her. She would blame herself, and Holly could never allow that. And in any case, what chance would she have in a court of law? She was a foreigner, practically penniless, and he belonged to one of the wealthiest families in Paris. He could afford the best lawyers in town.

And then came the most painful question of all: had she encouraged him in any way? Had she voluntarily or involuntarily let him believe that she would be willing to go along with his sex games? She had allowed him to play the dominant role in their relationship. She had spent a romantic evening with him, she had let him spend large sums of money on her, she had drunk more champagne than she could take, and then she had gone back with him to his apartment of her own free will. What had she expected? Seen in that light, she had only herself to blame.

Unexpectedly the taxi came to a halt and Holly saw that they had reached the street outside Arlette's home. She stared in dismay at the reading on the taxi meter. She had no idea how much money she had with her. She opened her bag and felt a surge of relief as her fingers closed round a fifty-franc note. As she pulled it out, something blue came with it and fell to the floor. She handed the money to the driver, got out and slammed the car door. He did not wait to see her pass through the gates into the courtyard. It was not often he was given fifteen francs as a tip and he was afraid that this passenger might ask for the change after all. He pulled away from the kerb at once and drove off into the night, taking Flo's letter with him.

FIFTEEN

On Arlette's return from Milan the following day, Holly wondered whether she should plead a headache and stay in her room. Sooner or later Arlette would want to know about her evening with Julien and she dreaded having to face her questions. When they finally met, she need not have worried. Arlette was so full of enthusiasm for the fabrics she has seen in Italy that their conversation was largely of a professional nature. Holly gave her a brief description of the dinner with Julien's colleagues from the bank. In typical French fashion Arlette wished to be told the menu in detail, but otherwise seemed satisfied with Holly's perfunctory replies to her enquiries. Holly made no mention of the visit to the nightclub and gave no impression that Julien's behaviour had been anything less than impeccable during her absence.

Her greatest fear was that they would meet again. Arlette was his aunt by marriage and frequently invited him to dinner. Holly's whole being revolted at the thought that she might have to speak to him. Sitting down at the same table would be unbearable. She did not even want to be in the same city. She was now desperate to go back to England as soon as possible. She must leave Paris at once. There was no alternative.

Spurred on by her anguish, that morning she had been to the Gare du Nord to enquire about train times and ticket prices. The sight of trains bound for the channel ports, English newspapers on the stands, and British travellers thronging the platforms had intensified her longing to escape.

Today she would write to Flo, she decided. It might ease the pain in her heart to tell her closest friend about the terrible happenings of the past night. Flo should be the first person to know that she was going back to England. The most difficult part would follow; she would have to inform Arlette of the decision she had made. The best time would be in the evening after dinner. No guests were expected and they would be alone together. But how would she tell Arlette, who treated her like a daughter, without hurting her? The kind Frenchwoman would feel deeply distressed by her sudden decision to leave, but if told the truth, she would blame herself for having encouraged the liaison with Julien. Holly hoped that she could somehow find enough plausible reasons to explain her sudden departure without having to mention him.

After dinner that evening Arlette sat down in front of the fire in the salon. She glanced up at Holly, who was standing at the window staring down into the courtyard below, quiet, almost morose, her vivacious sparkle gone like a snuffed-out candle. Arlette's practised eye took in the superb cut of Holly's black trouser suit, perfection in tailoring that combined a flawless appearance with an ease of movement as yet practically unknown in women's fashion. For the hundredth time that day she smoothed the pencil skirt of her Chanel suit over her hips.

As if she had known that Arlette was thinking about her, Holly turned and came towards her, her clothes underlining the easy grace of her movements. Arlette patted the couch to indicate that she should sit down beside her and pulled a pattern book of Italian tweeds onto her lap. She flipped it open, fingering the swatches of cloth it contained.

"Chérie, just look at these textures, these colour combinations. Feel the softness of the fabrics – pure merino wool woven with cashmere with just a touch of silk. Nothing stiff or scratchy. Signor Montefiori and his wife have a small business, just outside Milan. Their family have been weavers for generations. They have secret recipes for the dyes to make these glorious colours."

She paused to finger a swatch of tweed. It had the richness of a chocolate truffle but was shot with hues of crimson and cinnamon which seemed to change colour as light fell on it from different angles. She laid it aside almost reverently before she continued. "Signora Montefiori designs the fabrics. She has such a brilliant eye. So far they have been supplying the great houses, Dior, Chanel, Balenciaga, Balmain, but now they want to start a label of their own as well – a new twice-yearly collection for young women of today, based on perfectly cut trousers and skirts with matching jackets and coats, all in the finest, softest materials. The working title for the new line is 'Grazia', which means 'grace' or 'elegance' in Italian. I'd like you to submit a selection of your designs to the Montefioris, my dear. I'm absolutely sure that ideas like yours are just what they are looking for."

"Me?" Holly asked incredulously. She could not believe her ears. "But I'm not a trained fashion designer or anything like it. Surely . . ."

Arlette immediately put a stop to her protests. "An established designer with his or her own style is just what they want to avoid. Don't you see, Holly? They are after something really innovative. Something that hasn't been done before. Something created for the life that young women lead today, and who better to design such clothes than a young woman herself?" She leaned forward earnestly. "Ma chère, this is your chance. I told you it would come and I want you to take it. I'm convinced you can do it."

Holly was speechless, too thrilled to reply, but her eyes gave Arlette the answer she was hoping for. This was the opportunity of a lifetime. The silvery chimes of the little clock on the mantelpiece striking midnight found them both on their knees on the Aubusson carpet. Holly's designs of the last months littered the floor in concentric circles around them. Scraps of fabric were pinned to particular ones, some were crossed out and altered, others crumpled and rejected.

Arlette yawned delicately. "It's late, ma chère." She climbed wearily to her feet and looked down at the black and white sketches strewn around, standing out against the faded colours of the rug. "But there is such potential here, such talent. I'm sure you could get a portfolio together – with some new ideas as well, of course. Then we could send everything to Milan within, say, the next three to four weeks?"

"That's not long, but I think I can do it." Holly rose stiffly and stretched her aching back. "Will you be needing me in the office this week?"

"No, I'll be able to manage without you. You stay here and get as much work done as you possibly can," Arlette said generously, smiling. "After all, I've already sung your praises to Signor Montefiori. He'll be wanting to see some results. And I don't want him to be disappointed," she added with a teasing twinkle in her eye.

Holly ran her fingers through her hair. The enormity of the chance she was being offered was beginning to dawn on her at last. She drew a deep breath and looked Arlette in the eye. "I'll do my best," she said simply.

When Arlette had gone upstairs, Holly went to the window once more and looked out into the darkness below. She thought of her letter to Flo, still lying unfinished on the desk in her room upstairs. She had been going to post it in the morning. What should she do now?

She turned and looked at her work spread out on the carpet. She would never get a chance like this again. Should she really pass it up and return to England? She would be a fool if she did – and anyway she was only postponing her departure by a few weeks. She could complete this assignment and still be back in England in the summer.

The days went by. Holly worked without stopping, even taking her meals in her room. She had to convince the Italians that her ideas were the ones that would enhance their wonderful fabrics and embody the new line they envisaged. The deeper she immersed herself in her work, the easier it was for her to block out the appalling recollection of the night in Julien's apartment. She put all her efforts into completing her sketches, refusing to let the painful images of that horrifying occasion enter her head. But at night she had no control over her thoughts, and the memories returned to torment her. Julien's eyes rose before her and she heard his mocking laughter once again. Often she woke suddenly to find herself sitting upright in bed, shaking with fear, and it would be almost dawn before she fell into an uneasy sleep from which she rose unrefreshed, to begin working again the next day.

Arlette noted Holly's hollow cheeks and the signs of tiredness round her eyes. She said nothing, but instructed Madame Tourbie to send up regular trays piled with nourishing and appetising food, most of which, she noted with regret, came back down to the kitchen barely touched.

It was early one evening in June when Arlette tapped lightly on the door of Holly's room. Several weeks had passed since she had suggested the project and Holly was on her knees putting the finishing touches to the designs for her presentation.

"Ma chère, you work like a horse and live like a recluse," Arlette laughed, carefully sifting through the thick white sheets of paper which littered every available surface in the tiny room. "Oh là là," she said, shrugging her shoulders in a gesture of appreciation. "Mon Dieu, these designs are really magnifiques." She stood motionless, gazing down at the drawings, the be-ringed finger on one perfectly manicured hand tracing the lines on them almost reverently. "Holly, these are brilliant, fantastiques! I must admit, they are better than I ever imagined, and I was expecting a lot – but these . . ." As if lost for words, Arlette continued to gaze at the papers that lay scattered before her.

Holly sighed and rose wearily from her desk. She looked exhausted but satisfied and was pleased with the compliment. "This is the best I can do. It's up to Signor Montefiori to decide now. We can send the portfolio off to Italy in the morning."

"We'll send it by courier." Arlette bestowed a sparkling smile on her young protégée. "Ma chère, this calls for a celebration! Change out of those trousers, get dressed up and join us tonight. Maurice and Julien are coming to pick us up at nine. We are going to try out a new restaurant which le Tout-Paris says is absolument merveilleux. And you are marvellous too, my dear. You must come with us this evening and we shall have a wonderful dinner and drink lots of champagne to your future success."

"Oh no, Arlette. I'd rather not . . . " Holly searched her mind desperately for an adequate reason to prevent the meeting she dreaded, one that would not hurt this woman whom she was increasingly beginning to see less as an employer and more as a friend. "I'm so sorry, but I'd only spoil your evening. I'm feeling tired and I've got a headache." She spoke convincingly because the excuse that she had intended was the truth. Now that her presentation was complete, she was so exhausted that waves of giddiness seemed about to engulf her.

Arlette did not give in so easily. "Chérie," she pleaded. "We have seen nothing of you for so long. Julien told me on the phone today that he has almost forgotten how beautiful you are. Why, it's nearly a month since he last took you out. Please don't disappoint us. You must come with . . ."

Holly's blood all of a sudden seemed to freeze in her veins. The rest of Arlette's words were lost in a buzz of thoughts that crowded into her brain. It was not just the mention of his name which stunned her. A far greater fear seized her by the throat, choking her. Very firmly, knowing that she must seem brusque and impolite, even rude, she hustled Arlette out of the room and simply closed the door in her face.

Alone at last she rushed to find her shoulder bag. Rummaging through its various compartments she pulled out a battered leather-bound diary and leafed through it, hardly daring to breathe. She could feel her heart pounding against her ribs. One, two, three, four – she scanned the pages. Almost four weeks had passed since the evening she had done everything to forget. She had been so deeply immersed in her Italian project that she had failed to notice that she had missed her period.

A cold sweat broke out on her forehead. The nausea she had been feeling so often of late, the attacks of dizziness, the tautness of her breasts – everything fell into place. She knew without any shadow of doubt that she was expecting a child, a child from a man she despised, a child that had been conceived by a criminal act of violence. The fact imploded in her brain, cutting out all rational thought. She was overwhelmed with a sickening sense of horror. She felt nothing but disgust at the thought of bearing a child by the man she hated: disgust and naked fear.

She sat down on the edge of the bed in anguish, shivering with shock. She had been so horrified by Julien's behaviour on that terrible evening that she had never, even for a single moment, thought of the consequences it might lead to. She had been so intent on blotting him out of her mind that she had never considered she might become pregnant. Pregnant! The word alone filled her with horror. She was overwhelmed by a wave of revulsion; she was bearing the child of a man who had attacked and raped her.

She heard the sound of a car pulling up on the gravel in the courtyard below. She rushed in panic to the window and glanced down to see Julien's black Porsche drawing to a halt outside. As she watched, aghast, he jumped out and bounded nimbly up the stone steps that led to the entrance. He looked upwards, glancing in the direction of the window where she stood, and she drew back instantly. The very sight of him filled her with loathing. She had to escape.

There was no time to collect her coat or her bag. She had to be gone before he entered the apartment. She ran down the staircase to the floor below. There she opened a window leading onto the fire-escape and clambered out. One by one she scrambled down the flights of iron steps to the ground floor. She left the building through the tradesmen's entrance at the back from where she reached the anonymity of the street.

How far and how long did she walk that evening? She never noticed at the time and later on she could not say where she had been. All she knew was that she passed through familiar and unfamiliar streets, sometimes turning back on herself, never knowing where she was going. When at last she found herself beside the Seine, darkness had set in and the warmth of the evening had turned into the chill of night. She made her way along the bank until she came to the Pont Neuf. At its side, stone steps led down towards the water.

She stood on the bridge, staring down at the black, fast-flowing river. The wooden stands of the bouquinistes, the booksellers along its banks, were closed and locked. The last of the illuminated bateaux-mouches had long since slid past on its final journey. The students and lovers who sat on the benches during the day had gone to be together elsewhere. Even the clochards who sometimes slept under the bridge had found a warmer, better place to spend the night.

She was alone.

Slowly she started to descend the stone steps that led down to the water. She wanted to be near it. She saw how dark and cool it looked, how quickly it swirled away under the bridge. It would be so easy to go with it, to be drawn into one of those black vortexes and disappear into nothingness. She sat down on the bottom step, oblivious of its slimy green coating, and stared. A cold rationality overcame her that surprised her. If she were brave enough to jump, what would that solve? Death would have no reason, serve no purpose. It could never be an end in itself but simply a negation of life, and even at this moment she knew that her will to live was stronger than her despair.

She rose and mounted the steps again. At the top she noticed a lighted café on a street corner opposite. Through the window she could see that it was empty. A solitary waiter was behind the bar, polishing glasses. If he was surprised to see a young woman come in on her own after midnight, he did not show it. When Holly told him that she had lost her purse and asked if she could use the phone, he pushed it wordlessly towards her.

"Hello, Arlette? It's me, Holly."

"Holly, Mon Dieu! Ma petite, where are you? We have been so worried about you. Are you alright? Where are you? What has happened?" Arlette sounded frantic.

"Don't worry, I'm alright," Holly began, anxious to allay her worst fears at once. "Are you alone?"

"Of course not," Arlette replied rather crossly. "Julien is here with me. He wouldn't hear of leaving until we found out where you are. We were just about to phone the police or the hospital. Where are you? I can send Julien over in his car to pick you up."

"No, please. Look, Arlette. I can't explain on the phone, but I have to see you alone. Absolutely alone. Julien must not be there. Please tell him to go home. I'll be back with you in about fifteen minutes, but I have to see you alone," she repeated.

Arlette adopted a warning tone. "I hope this isn't some sort of joke."

"Believe me, Arlette, I have never been so serious in my life."

Holly put the phone down. She made her way back to the apartment quickly. The air was cold and it was raining heavily when she arrived. A glance inside the courtyard confirmed that Julien's car had gone. Arlette must have been watching from the window because as soon as Holly stepped out of the lift she flung the door to the apartment open, rushed out and took her in her arms, only to draw back in horror.

"Mon Dieu, my dear child, you are all wet. Outside without a coat in this weather! And your hands, they're frozen. Come in and get warm before you catch a dreadful cold!" She ushered Holly into the salon where she threw another log onto the fire, sat Holly down on one of the sofas and pulled a rug round her shoulders. "Shall I make you a warm drink? Some tea, un chocolat? Or brandy perhaps? A glass of cognac?"

"Please no," Holly begged. "I'll be fine. Just sit down here with me so I can tell you everything."

Arlette did not have to be asked a second time. She sat down beside her and waited expectantly, her whole bearing showing deep anxiety and concern.

Holly took a deep breath. Telling her story to Arlette was not going to be easy. What she had to say would hurt her and shock her, but she knew she had no alternative. While she spoke, Arlette's eyes never left her face. At times they blazed with anger, at times they filled with tears. "I blame myself," she said at last. "I should never have let you go out alone with Julien."

Holly almost laughed aloud despite the seriousness of the situation. "Arlette, je t'en prie! I'm twenty-two! I'm old enough to look after myself. Or at least I should be," she added. "You warned me what he was like. It was my fault that I didn't take you seriously. I . . ." Her voice faltered. "I tried to play with fire and I got my fingers burned. I must have drunk too much wine and champagne that evening. I should never have gone with him to his apartment. I don't know why I did. It was as if I somehow lost control of what I was doing. I don't know why."

Arlette's face darkened. "I'm afraid I think I do," she said grimly. "You know that Julien spent the last years working in the Far East?" Holly nodded, wondering what this fact had to do with herself. "My dear, he did not go there of his own choice. A woman colleague of his had accused him of trying to rape her. She said that he had slipped something into her drink. Julien told us that she was lying, trying to get him out of the way because they were rivals for the same position in the bank, and of course my husband and I believed him. After all, he was Henri's nephew. The woman got the post and Julien was shipped off to Singapore. The bank could not allow the faintest whiff of scandal, you see, and the whole thing got covered up." She took Holly's hand in hers. "I've never thought about it since, until tonight. He must have used the same trick with you."

"What does it matter now? We'll never know."

"You are sure about the baby?"

Holly nodded. "I haven't been to see a doctor yet, but all the signs are there." They sat in silence, each staring ahead into the flames.

Arlette pressed her hand. "I know of a very good clinic in Montparnasse where you could go. I'll pay for the . . . I'll pay, if you don't want to keep the child."

Holly sighed. "I'll pay you back when I can." She ignored Arlette's gesture of refusal. "Why would I want to keep it? When I think of . . . of him, and what he did to me . . . and when I think that the baby is his . . ." Exhaustion finally took over and she collapsed in tears.

Arlette called Marie and together they helped Holly to her room where they put her to bed like a child. Left alone in the darkness she closed her eyes tightly, trying in vain to dispel her thoughts. How could a baby be conceived by such a terrible act of violence? Another act of violence must follow to get rid of it. It was the only way.

SIXTEEN

Arlette took charge. After a gynaecologist had confirmed that Holly was pregnant, she made an appointment at a private clinic in Montparnasse where the termination – she delicately used that word rather than the term 'abortion' – would be discreetly carried out. Holly went for a preliminary examination during which very few questions were asked and the date was fixed for the Wednesday of the next week.

Hour by hour the intervening time dragged past. The weekend came and went. Holly and Arlette spent it quietly at home. In a stormy interview, Arlette told Julien in the plainest of terms that he was never to come near the apartment and that neither she nor Holly ever wished to see him again. His protestations that he loved Holly, that she had consented to their affair, even encouraged him, went unheeded. Eventually he drove off in anger and the two women were left together, outwardly in each other's company but inwardly alone, each with her own thoughts and self-recriminations.

In the mornings the bouts of nausea steadily increased, as if her whole body were rebelling against the seed that had been planted in it. In the evenings Arlette had tempting dishes prepared to encourage Holly to eat, but herself set a poor example. During dinner they both avoided the subject that was uppermost on their minds, conversation became stilted or dried up completely and Holly escaped as soon as possible to the sanctuary of her room, unable to think, numb with shock and worry. When, in the early hours, she fell into a troubled sleep at last, there was a big black hole in her heart where her feelings should have been.

When Monday came, she awoke feeling worse than ever. She was sitting up in bed, trying to avoid the sight of a tray of tea and toast which Marie had placed beside her, when the door flew open and Arlette rushed in without knocking. Holly stared at her in blank amazement. It was not just unheard of for Arlette to be up so early in the morning, but to appear en déshabillé was totally out of character. Barefoot, her hair down, her negligée flying open to reveal her nightdress, she had obviously leapt straight out of bed. She was waving a telegram excitedly in one hand.

"Chérie, I am so happy for you! It has happened! I knew it would! I can hardly believe it!" The illogicality of her words made the situation only more baffling. She flung her arms round Holly and kissed her soundly on both cheeks.

"Look, ma chère, just look at this," she cried, flapping the telegram in front of Holly's face so that it was impossible for her to do so.

Holly's curiosity overcame her nausea. "Arlette, what is it? What's happened?"

"The Montefioris love your designs! They want to use them – and not just that. Oh Holly, they want you – and only you – to design their next collections for them as well – two collections a year! Of course the collections won't be large, but they want daywear for business and leisure – all with the young woman of today in mind! Isn't that wonderful – just fantastic – merveilleux! " Running out of epithets in English, she lapsed into her mother tongue.

The lines on the telegram danced before Holly's eyes. The Montefioris wanted to discuss the terms of the contract. She was to fly to Milan at their expense as soon as it was convenient.

"But they can't want me! I mean, I'm not a trained fashion designer. I'm not qualified. I've never graduated from college."

"College? Pouf!" The dramatic gesture sent hairpins flying. "What can you learn there? A lot of theory that could ruin your talent." Arlette's voice dropped to take on a note of profound intensity. "*This* is your chance. It will open the door to your career. Opportunities like this don't come twice. Turn it down and you will regret it for the rest of your days!" Then, embarrassed either by the violence of her words or a sudden awareness of the state of her appearance, she pulled her negligée tightly around herself and rushed out of the room.

Holly read the telegram once more. Every word that Arlette had said was true. It was the chance of a lifetime, a dream come true. Her emotions had rocketed from misery and despair to joy and excitement within seconds. She could not believe it. She had to calm down and think clearly. What she needed was to talk it over with someone. Flo, with her wonderful common sense, had never seemed so far away. Then she remembered her grandfather. She had been so busy working on the Montefiori portfolio that she had not visited him of late. At the thought of her only relation, she felt calmer. It would be good to see him again. She pulled the breakfast tray towards her.

Guy de Valmont was pruning roses in the front garden of his home when she arrived. His face creased into a smile at the sight of her and he came forward to embrace her, arms outstretched, tall and upright with an almost military bearing. He was wearing corduroy trousers, a checked shirt with the sleeves rolled up over his tanned sinewy forearms, and a cotton sun hat that he removed to mop his brow with a large white handkerchief.

"Bonjour, ma petite-fille." He kissed her. His whole being radiated the life and warmth that had been so lacking on her first visit. "Isn't it a lovely day? Summer is on the way. Do you know, I heard a cuckoo in the Bois this morning. Come and sit down with me so we can enjoy a glass of lemonade together." He led her round the back of the house to a wooden bench under a cherry tree heavy with blossom.

Holly sat in the sunshine until he returned with two glasses and a jug of juice with cubes of ice floating in it, not a fizzy drink as she had expected, but made from fresh lemons.

"Marie-Joséphine makes this. She lives in the flat above mine. She insists that I don't drink enough. She is very good to me. Santé, ma petite." They clinked their glasses. "Now tell me all your news." He leant back, looking at her fondly.

Holly told him about the offer the Montefioris had made. He nodded appreciatively. "You've done very well, my dear. I am proud of you. You must have inherited your father's talent. I will show you some of his drawings and paintings when we go indoors." He looked into her eyes. "But there is more, isn't there?" His face softened and his voice became gentle. "You have brought such wonderful news, but there is something else, isn't there? Your father used to look like that when he was unhappy. Something is troubling you. Do you think you could tell me about it, my dear?"

Her self-control snapped and she burst into tears. The numbness of the past days was gone and the pain swept through her. Between huge sobs she told him everything, how Julien had raped her, and about the child she was expecting. "And on Wednesday," she finished, "I have an appointment at a clinic to . . . " She broke down again.

Wordlessly he took her in his arms and let her weep. When her sobs subsided, he handed her his big handkerchief. "It has all happened so fast, my dear. Are you sure you have thought this over carefully? Is an abortion what you really want?"

She shuddered. "I can't bear the thought of him and what he did to me, but . . ." She broke down again.

"It is not the child's fault. You must not forget, part of this child is you. It cannot be blamed for the way it was conceived. Even if you kill the child, you cannot undo the wrong that this man has done to you. The memory will always be there."

"But every time I look at the child, it will remind me of him."

He shook his head. "I think not, my dear. A child is the most precious possession there is. Perhaps one only realizes just how precious when one has lost it." He wiped his eyes before he spoke again. "Think how your own mother, Elizabeth, must have felt when she realized that she was expecting a child, having lost the man she loved. In spite of all the difficulties she had to face she gave you the gift of life."

Holly stayed silent, not trusting herself to speak.

"The decision is yours," he continued, "but I will accept whatever you decide and I will do everything I can to help you." He rose to his feet. "Come with me now."

He led her inside the house. In the sitting-room he pulled a large folder out from behind the sideboard. Inside there were pencil sketches, drawings in charcoal, or pen and ink, and further paintings, some of which were unfinished. Most were country scenes or studies of still life, but there were several portraits of a beautiful woman whom Holly recognized as Geneviève, her grandmother.

"These are wonderful." She looked through them, turning them over one by one. "My work is nothing compared to this."

"Your talent is different," he said simply. "No child is the same as its parent. No one knows what qualities a child will inherit." He returned the sheets carefully, reverently, to the folder. "And now I will show you more."

He led the way out of his apartment into the hallway and up some stairs. They climbed two flights, past other flats, until they came to the top floor. There he pulled a key from his pocket and unlocked a door.

Holly found herself inside a converted loft. Despite its sloping walls it was large and spacious. Light poured into the room from mansard windows on both sides. It was completely empty. In one corner there was a makeshift kitchen. Their feet echoed on the wooden floorboards as they crossed to two doors which led off the main area, one to a second, much smaller room, the other to a tiny bathroom.

"I don't want to influence your decision at all," he said, "but if you wish to stay in Paris and you cannot continue living with your friend Arlette, you can live here. The last tenant has just moved out and left the key with me. The rent is low. I know the landlord well, so I could arrange for you to have it if you wanted. Say nothing now. Think about what I have said, and always remember, ma chère petite-fille, that you are not alone." He embraced her wordlessly as she said goodbye.

When she returned home, Arlette had gone to the office. A note on the hall table announced that she would not be back till late that night. Holly went to her room and it was Tuesday evening before she met Arlette again. They shared an early, largely silent meal, but this time Holly did not rush off afterwards. She followed Arlette into the salon where the Frenchwoman watched her anxiously. She noted Holly's reddened eyes and pale skin flushed with nervousness, as if she were dreading her appointment at the clinic the next morning.

How shall I begin? Holly wondered. An abortion had always seemed the obvious solution; they had never discussed any alternative. How shall I begin to tell her that I've decided to keep this child after all? Will she understand that I want it to live, just as my mother allowed me to live? It's a part of me, my son or my daughter, the only family except Grandfather that I have in the world. It's not an object I can throw away. Not after all I have lost.

It was as if she had spoken the words aloud. Arlette was staring straight at her. "Holly, my dear, are you certain about tomorrow?" It was a question she had never voiced until now.

Holly took a deep breath. "I'm not going to the clinic, Arlette." She tried to keep her voice steady. "I've decided that I'm going to keep the baby."

In an instant Arlette's arms were around her, her eyes brimming with tears. "Are you sure?"

"I made up my mind last night. I thought you'd be upset when I told you."

"Upset? Oh Holly, how could I be upset? I'm so happy!"

"Happy?" This time it was Holly's turn to be amazed.

"So happy! I know what it is to lose a child. I didn't dare suggest it but I prayed that you would keep the baby. It will be hard for you, but I will help you in every way I can. Believe me, my dear, Julien's family are not all like he is. He has a terrible streak in his character like his father had, but his mother, my husband's sister, was such a wonderful person. She died when he was ten. Perhaps it will be a boy like my Henri or a little girl like my darling Virginie. A child in my home again. Oh Holly, that would be wonderful."

"Arlette, it's so kind of you to offer but I can't stay here. We both know that. You have your position in society to consider. This is no place for an unmarried mother with an illegitimate child." She quickly interrupted Arlette's protests. It would be better for her to have somewhere of her own, she said. Excitedly she told her about the loft in her grandfather's house.

Arlette was delighted. "That's the perfect solution! You'll have space there to work and room for the baby as well. Your grandfather is there, and I will come as often as I can to see you. And you know you will always be welcome here." She reached out and took both of Holly's hands in her own.

"I know," Holly said gratefully.

The barrier that had stood between them for so long had been breached at last. Arlette brought out an album of photographs of her husband and her little daughter. As they looked at the pictures together she spoke openly of the love and happiness she had lost. Holly saw how deeply she had suffered.

"But I have my memories," she said, closing the book at last. "No one can take them from me, and there comes a time when one must look to the future, not to the past, and move forward." Holly wondered whether Arlette was going to mention her relationship with Maurice, but her next words referred to her.

"Holly, what was it that made you change your mind about the baby?"

There was a long pause before Holly answered. She felt that she owed Arlette an answer, but despite the intimacy of their conversation it was one which she could not give.

"I'm sorry, Arlette. Something happened a long time ago. In England." Her eyes filled with tears. "One day I'll be able to tell you about it, I promise. But not now, not yet."

There was a finality in her voice that made Arlette want to reach out to comfort her again, but at that moment the little clock on the mantelpiece chimed ten and Holly rose abruptly.

"Excuse me a minute, Arlette. It's not too late. If you don't mind, there are a couple of phone calls I have to make."

She went into the adjoining study. First she dialled the clinic and cancelled her appointment for the morning. Then she rang the airport and booked a flight to Milan.

SEVENTEEN

Paris, June 1969

It was Flo's first visit to Paris. Now that she was teaching in York she had managed to save enough to make the trip. Their reunion had been a joyful one. In fact they had hardly stopped talking since the moment Flo had stepped out of the train at the Gare du Nord. Holly was looking forward to showing her the beauties of the city, but undeniably its greatest attraction was sitting on the floor in front of them. Holly could not resist teasing her oldest friend.

"Flo! Have you come all this way to play with Rose or to get a wedding dress?"

"She's just so gorgeous, I can't take my eyes off her. Oh Holly, if Mike and I ever have a little girl, I want her to be just like yours."

"Well, make sure you get married first! It makes life a lot easier."

Although she was joking, she could not prevent a serious note from creeping into her voice. Life was often hard, living alone with no regular income and a child to support, but Rose made everything worthwhile. She gazed at the little girl sitting on the blanket, examining a toy dog Flo had brought her, turning it over and over in her chubby hands. Despite her tender age of sixteen months, she seemed to enjoy being the centre of attention, fixing her admirers with eyes as green as deep mountain lakes. When her rosy-cheeked face crowned by a circle of unruly black curls broke into a smile, it was like the sun emerging through clouds. That this lovely child, with her almost mystic Celtic looks, was the baby she had not wanted – the thought was almost too painful to contemplate. What would her life be without Rose?

For the moment there were more pressing questions to answer. What would Flo say when she saw the wedding dress Holly had designed and made to the measurements her friend had sent? Would she like it? Would it suit her? What if it did not fit? At Christmas Flo and Mike would be getting married. Flo was going to move from York to teach at Ainsley school, Mike would take over his father's farm and the two would live in the dales farmhouse. As soon as her friend had written to tell her of their engagement, Holly had decided that Flo's gown would be her wedding present.

She felt more nervous about this fitting than if she were working in a famous fashion house. She lifted the dress from the tailor's dummy and placed it carefully over her friend's head.

She need not have worried.

"I can't believe it's me. Pinch me so I know I'm not dreaming." Flo was staring entranced at her reflection in the long mirror in Holly's studio. She turned slowly. The soft folds of silk gently traced the generous curves of her body, while its pure white sheen enhanced the glow of her English-rose complexion.

Her brows drawn in concentration, Holly made a tiny adjustment to the set of the shoulders. Several other minor alterations were necessary, but she was delighted with her creation. No frills, no fuss, no glitter: just glamour. Nothing spoilt the simple lines of her design. The deep v-shaped neckline, the long tapering sleeves, and the slightly dropped waistline of the bodice lengthened Flo's figure, and combined with the sweeping train of the skirt created a slimming effect and added an impression of the height she lacked.

"I've never felt like this in my whole life, I feel absolutely beautiful! Oh Holly, it's so wonderful. How can I ever thank you?"

Flo's shining eyes gave Holly the answer. She looked up and smiled at her friend in the mirror. "By being the happiest woman in the world on your wedding day," she announced. She put the last pins in place and lifted the dress over Flo's head.

Flo struggled back into her shirt and jeans. "You will come to the wedding, won't you?" she asked anxiously. "You just have to. Mike specially asked me to tell you how much he wants you to be there as well. Promise you'll come, and bring Rose as well."

"I'll do my best, really I will." Holly avoided her friend's eyes as she put the gown back onto the dummy. She longed to return to the moors again, and attending the wedding of her two oldest friends at the same time was more than she dared hope for at present. Money was more than tight and travelling as far as the north of England seemed like an impossible dream. "I'll see what I can do," she said firmly, bringing the subject to a close. "Let's go back down now and have some tea."

Rose ran over to them and Flo bent down to scoop her into her arms. Casting a last delighted glance at the dress, she followed Holly out of the attic loft that served as her studio. They made their way to the ground floor flat which was now her home. As they entered, Holly thought lovingly of Guy de Valmont. Six months after Rose's birth she had come down from the loft where she lived and worked, to find him sitting in the sun on his favourite bench under the cherry tree. He had looked at peace, as if he had fallen asleep, but a sudden stroke had taken his life. Even now sadness filled her at the memory of the grandfather she had found, only to lose again so soon. Though the time they had spent together had been short, a bond had grown between them. She was happy that he had lived long enough to see Rose, but she knew that even his great-grandchild had not assuaged the pain of losing his beloved wife and son. She hoped they were together again now.

After his funeral, when the ground floor flat was to be let again, she had decided to take it on as well. Living in the loft was manageable while Rose was a baby, but Holly had seen that, as soon as she began to move around, it was going to be impossible. She herself did not mind living and working in one space since she had virtually no private life, but with a lively toddler to care for, she had realised it would be difficult to cope. The rooms under the roof were hot and airless in the Parisian summer, whereas the flat downstairs included the use of the shady garden. Paying two rents put a severe strain on her budget, but she managed to scrape by.

They entered the flat. Holly had painted the rooms white and furnished them sparsely, combining pieces from her grandfather with bargains she found at the flea market. Arlette had offered to help and, though Holly had wanted neither money nor anything from her luxurious apartment, she had been happy to accept the gift of some simple furniture for the nursery. Flo laid Rose down for her afternoon nap in her little white bed with its rosebud-patterned covers, while Holly went into the kitchen. When she came back with two mugs of tea and a plate of English biscuits, they took them into the sitting-room.

She found Flo staring at the portrait of Geneviève de Valmont. Holly treasured the painting of her grandmother and had left it together with her father's watercolours in their original places on the walls.

"Holly, I can't believe it. She looks exactly like you. The likeness is absolutely amazing."

"I know. It was when I saw that picture that I knew for the first time who I really was. I have a few pieces of her jewellery, too. They mean so much to me, I'd never sell them. One day they'll belong to Rose. Poor Grandfather, that was all he had to leave us."

Flo looked round the little room. It was elegant in its simplicity, with a delicate, feminine touch. "This is home for you now, isn't it?"

Holly nodded. "Yes, it's my home and Rose's. Where else can we go? I have my work here, so this is where I have to be."

Flo could hear the melancholy in her voice. "I can imagine how hard it's been for you." The blue eyes that met Holly's brown ones seemed to melt with sympathy. "Oh Holly, I was so sad and worried about you when you told me what happened that night with Julien. I never dreamt you'd keep the baby. I don't know whether I would have had the courage to do that."

There was a short silence as Holly sipped her tea reflectively before she spoke. "I don't really think it was courage at all. More the opposite in fact. There was suddenly just no way I could have gone through with an abortion. Not after . . ." She could not go on.

"You poor thing. It must have been awful having a baby here all on your own."

"Grand-père was a tremendous help and Arlette has been fantastic. She's even kept me on as her personal assistant at the magazine. That and the money I get from the Montefiori designs is what Rose and I have to live on." Her voice wavered slightly. "I couldn't have gone back to England. I had no work there, not enough money to go to college and support Rose, nowhere to live and," she paused imperceptibly, "I couldn't have faced meeting Nick again."

"Oh Holly, do you still think about Nick Ranleigh? Surely not after all this time?"

Her friend's expression gave her the answer.

"You mean, there's been no one ever since?"

"No one who has meant anything to me. I've tried hard, but it's no use." She let herself ask the question which had been on her lips since Flo's arrival. "Have you heard anything about him, where he is or what he's doing? Is he married?"

"I met Georgina on the street in York just a month or so ago. She's teaching at the convent school there and engaged to marry a solicitor. She told me that Nick had left London to do post-graduate training in plastic surgery, but she didn't say where. I'm sure she would have said something if he'd been married. She asked after you, by the way."

"Did she?" Holly wondered how much about her present situation would get passed on to Nick.

"I told her you were doing very well in Paris, making a name for yourself in the fashion world, but I didn't go into any more detail." Holly could have kissed her for her discretion. "But Holly, don't you think it's time to put all that behind you? You have so much going for you here."

Dear Flo, sensible and down-to-earth as ever.

"You're right," Holly admitted. "Things are starting to turn out really well."

"Tell me more." Flo was curled up on one end of the sofa, her feet tucked under her. Holly was reminded of the confidences they used to share in her bedroom in the farmhouse. They seemed to have taken place in another world.

"Where shall I start?"

"Start at the beginning."

Holly laughed. "I suppose the beginning was when Rose was born. The birth was awful, mainly because I was on my own in this French hospital, hooked up to all these machines and monitors with an ancient midwife yelling at me in French."

"Don't!" Flo rolled her eyes in horror. "When I have a baby, I certainly won't come here to have it!"

"Well, I suppose it was just me, not the hospital's fault. It's not easy having a baby by someone you hate. When the pains got bad, it was like being raped all over again."

Flo's laughter ceased. "You poor dear," she said softly.

"That was the bad bit. Once that was over, I adored Rose the minute I saw her. She made up for everything."

"Why did you call her Rose? It's a funny name for a baby born in February."

Holly smiled at the recollection. "It was Arlette who named her. She was my first and only visitor. She came to the hospital – she's always so beautifully groomed and elegant, you know – well, this time she appeared with no hat, no gloves, in a jacket that didn't match her skirt, holding this enormous bouquet of pink roses. She was so desperate to see the baby and so worried about me, she must have rushed off as soon as she got the news! When she took the baby into her arms, there were tears running down her face. She must have been remembering her own little daughter who was killed. All she could say was "une petite rose". She has been my little Rose ever since."

"What a lovely story!" Flo looked wistful.

"More than anything else in the world I want her to be

happy. I want her life to be like summer! Mine has often seemed like winter," Holly added, almost to herself.

"It must have been hard. How have you managed since Rose was born? How on earth have you coped with work and looking after a baby as well?"

"Arlette has been wonderful, almost like a grandmother really, though don't you dare tell her I said so because she is very conscious of her age even though she's only in her forties. But of course she lives quite a distance away so can't lend a hand all the time. She even helped me pay for my car so I can take Rose over to see her more easily. Then there was my grandfather, but he died soon after Rose was born and there's only so much you can ask a seventy-five-year-old man to do, even if it is his great-granddaughter! My main lifeline has been Marie-Joséphine. She used to look after my grandfather. She lives in the flat directly above this one with her husband, Salim. He's a cook in an Arab restaurant. They're wonderful people, so friendly and helpful, though Algerians don't have a very easy time in France these days. They've got three children of their own, so Rose has friends to play with as well. I don't know what I'd do without her."

As she finished speaking there was a knock on the door. "That'll be Marie-Jo now." Holly went to open it and came back with a woman of about their own age, dressed in a blue cotton caftan that ended to reveal sturdy brown legs and bare feet in open leather sandals. Holly introduced her visitor to Flo. Marie-Jo's strong white teeth parted in a wide smile. The sound of their voices woke Rose, and Marie-Jo was instantly at her bedside, lifting her out and cooing soft words in her native Arabic.

"I'll take her upstairs to my bunch and give them all their supper." Rose was nestling against Marie-Jo's shoulder with her thumb in her mouth. "Then I'll bring her back down and put her to bed. I'll stay here till you get back tonight. Salim's off duty so he can take care of our lot. We'll have a nice time together, won't we, Rose?"

The little girl seemed to welcome the prospect and clapped her hands. "Have a great night out with your friend!"

Marie-Jo flashed her broad smile at Holly again. "And don't rush back!"

Holly thanked her gratefully. She had been looking forward to this evening for weeks. It was rare that she was able to go out socially. It was not just looking after Rose that kept her at home; most days she had to work until late, often into the early hours of the morning. It was a heavy burden, but at eight o'clock, as the door of the flat snapped into its lock behind her, she felt liberated. Just for one night she was free from responsibilities, free to enjoy herself.

On an impulse she took Flo's arm and they were soon giggling like schoolgirls again as they headed for the Métro that would take them to the bright lights of the boulevards.

EIGHTEEN

Still in her pyjamas Flo padded barefoot into the kitchen. "Oh my head! I don't think we should have had that second bottle of red wine." She lowered herself gingerly onto a chair at the table where Holly was spooning cereal into Rose's open mouth. "Maybe if I sit here quietly without moving I might be able to survive the day."

Holly laughed. "Well, you were the one who ordered it. At least you'll have something to remember from your night out in Paris!"

"Oh Holly, it was so fantastic. You know, when I'm stuck in the farmhouse in the snow next winter, I'm going to remember it all. That gorgeous meal in that lovely little restaurant with the nice waiter! I'm sure tourists never get to see places like that. Then walking along the boulevards in the Latin quarter at midnight. There were so many people about – on the streets, in the cafés and in the bars. I can't wait to tell Mike about it."

"If you do, I wouldn't mention that discotheque in Saint-Germain where we ended up. He might not be so keen on the idea of you dancing with all those Frenchmen!"

"Did I?" Flo's blue eyes opened wide in feigned astonishment.

"You did. It took me all my strength to get you into the taxi." Holly shook her head in mock disapproval, but in fact she was delighted that Flo had enjoyed their evening out so much. The dinner, which Holly had insisted on paying for, the taxi fare and other expenses had torn a large hole in her budget for the month, but had been worth every franc. She could not remember when she had last felt so carefree. Her friend's visit was like a holiday for her.

"I could do with some tea," Flo announced, lifting Rose out of her high chair and cuddling her on her lap for a moment before the little girl struggled free and ran off to fetch her favourite toys. "Do you have some real tea made from tea leaves, not that awful stuff the French call 'tea' that's made from dried lime leaves, camomile, peppermint or something similarly vile? You know, the stuff that chimps drink on telly?"

Holly grinned and lifted the pot. "Already brewed." They sat in silence for a while, watching Rose play, enjoying each other's company.

"Holly," Flo began, "I'm having such a great time here but there's something I'd still like to see."

Holly looked up, surprised, wondering which sights her friend might want to visit that they had missed out.

"Of course. Where would you like to go?"

"You haven't shown me any of the clothes you've designed, except for my wedding dress, of course. I'd love to see more of your work."

"Really? I thought you might want to do some more sightseeing or go shopping today."

"I've already seen far more than I can remember and I haven't got the money for shopping. I'd much prefer to have a look at some of the work you do. If that's alright with you?"

"Sure, why not? We can start right here." Holly bent to scoop Rose into her arms. "Let's go upstairs to my studio."

Flo pretended to be horrified. "There is no way I'm going to look at Paris fashions in my Snoopy pyjamas! I've got enough complexes about my looks as it is! And I haven't taken my pill yet."

"You're on the pill?"

"Of course. Heavens, Holly, wake up! It's 1969! All the girls are on it nowadays. Maybe you should be too!" She scuttled off into the bathroom, then peeped mischievously round the door. "You never know! Just in case!"

Ten minutes later they climbed the stairs to the loft. Flo waited expectantly as Holly picked up a large portfolio, leafed through its contents and laid the sketches one by one on the large table in the centre of the studio. Flo said nothing while she moved around, studying them intently. Then she spoke. "I can't pretend to know much about fashion but these look fantastic to me."

Holly looked down at the drawings for the Montefioris' next spring collection. "These designs are for an Italian firm. They weave these gorgeous textiles. I've been working for them for over two years now, doing two collections a year. These will be part of their 1970 spring range." She fingered the swatches of fabric attached to each of the designs. Cool shades of blue, smoky grey and pale green seemed to dominate, but there were hues of coffee, apricot and cinnamon as well. Flo came to her side and touched the soft materials respectfully. Some were light tweeds with intermingling colours, often fine wool shot with silk, others as delicate as cotton voile and almost as transparent. Holly explained the sketches, often pointing out details which her friend's inexperienced eye would otherwise have missed.

"These coats and suits, the dresses, even the skirts and sweaters – everything's so young and up-to date, but at the same time so elegant," Flo sighed at last. "I've always admired Italian women for their sense of style, they are just sort of effortlessly chic, but anyone who's lucky enough to wear these clothes is going to look even better than they do. Everything matches so perfectly. Who's it all aimed at?"

"Women in their twenties or early thirties."

"And who have quite a lot of money, I should imagine!"

"Yes, I'm afraid so," Holly admitted regretfully. "The Grazia collection is very expensive. First there are the exclusive fabrics, then the garments are practically hand-made, and so far they have only been on sale in high-class boutiques in places like Rome, Milan, Zurich, St Moritz and so on, so you can imagine what the prices are like. Not the sort of clothes people like you and I are ever going to be able to afford. I'm a bit disappointed really."

"Why so?" Flo looked closely at her friend. "Did you expect something different?"

"Yes I did, in a way. The whole assignment hasn't really turned out as I thought it would. My basic idea is that young women of today need a new style of clothes for the life they lead, because it's so different from the life their mothers led. So they don't want what their mother wore – you know, daytime dresses, narrow jackets with tight skirts and all that. When I started on the collection, I had working women like us in mind who might want to splash out on something extra nice once in a while which would make them feel really good."

She gestured at the sketches lying on the table. "As you can see, the Montefioris have other ideas, which don't exactly coincide with mine. Obviously they want their gorgeous fabrics and colours to be used to full effect, so the whole collection has turned out to be far more feminine and luxurious than I originally intended. Of course I have to go along with them because I can't afford to lose the assignment, but I doubt whether the women who buy these pieces will have earned the money to pay for them themselves! They probably won't even need to work at all. It's far more likely to be their husbands or rich boyfriends who're footing the bill!"

"But I think your idea's wonderful. You mustn't lose sight of it."

Holly was already sweeping the papers on the table back into the folder. "I haven't," she grinned. She produced a second, larger portfolio, opened it and laid out another, completely different set of designs. At once Flo noted the stark contrast with the sketches of the previous collection. On each page no more than three or four bold black lines joined or crossed to create simple but powerful images. Flo felt rather than saw the impression of strength and movement which they imparted.

"Holly, *this* is you. These are brilliant."

Holly's eyes were shining. "This is what I've always wanted to design. Clothes for young women of today who really have to work for their living. They need clothes that make them look good and feel confident, clothes they can move about it, work in, travel in, clothes that let them compete with men but at the same time never forget they're a woman. They don't want to dress up to look like baby dolls, Russian peasants or something from the Arabian nights, and they can't, if they want to be taken seriously."

She pulled one of the designs towards her so that Flo could see it better. "This trouser suit is one of the basics. It's cut largely on the bias so that the wearer has complete freedom and ease of movement, but at the same time the lines make her look slim and elegant, even if she hasn't got a perfect figure."

"That's just what I need. I can never find anything in the shops like that. Either clothes are comfortable and then look like a sack on me, or they look good, in which case they are digging into me half the time."

Holly smiled. "This wouldn't. And it's not just the cut. The materials must be natural and top quality – superb wools, cottons and silks – because you can't create a beautiful garment from shoddy fabric. And most important of all, the workmanship has to be of the highest standard. No buttons that fall off, zips that get stuck, puckered seams, loose threads, drooping hems – nothing like that. The woman who wears my clothes has to be able to rely on them totally to see her through the whole day, simply because she's got more important things on her mind – her work, her leisure time, her partner, her family, whatever."

They looked together through the designs. Besides several versions of a trouser suit, both single- and double-breasted, there were jackets and trench coats and a range of pants and skirts. The collection was not large, but it all bore the same signature. "I thought the designs for the Montefioris were elegant but this beats everything," Flo sighed. "Couldn't you persuade the Italians to accept these instead?"

"They want the style I showed you before, the one which suits their extravagant fabrics. It's understandable. My designs don't need elaborate materials in fancy colours. The wearer that I've got in mind wants to wear basics – that's black, navy, grey, beige or white. She can always combine her suit or coat with a colourful top or accessories, but any more colour on the garment itself would interfere with the purity of the line."

Flo nodded. " I see what you mean, but if you can't get the

Montefioris to produce them, who will you get?"

Holly took a deep breath. "I've started to produce them myself, under my own label. If you want, you can come with me this afternoon and see how. And now," she said, putting the sketches back inside the folder, "it's such a gorgeous day and Paris is so lovely in June. Let's take Rose in her pushchair for a walk in the Luxembourg Gardens."

After an early lunch Holly and Flo left Rose asleep in Marie-Jo's care and set off in Holly's car across the city, travelling eastwards till they reached a part of Paris which Flo had not seen yet.

"This quarter is called the Marais," Holly explained as her ancient Citroën 2CV rattled over the cobbles of a narrow street lined with stone buildings so tall as to block out the sunlight. "It's one of the oldest parts of Paris. When the Louvre fortress was made into a royal palace, some of the nobles at court moved into the Marais and built themselves magnificent residences called 'hôtels', mainly for entertaining. Lots of the ones you see now date from the sixteenth or seventeenth centuries." She spotted a parking space and reversed into it smartly. "Some of them have been turned into museums or government offices, others are still more or less derelict, like this one."

The noise of the modern city had died away. Only the cries of children at a nearby playground broke the stillness. Holly looked up at the ancient building, huge and imposing with stone carving and iron-studded doors, now deserted and desolate. She envisaged it in its glory of so long ago: lights blazing at the windows, carriages bearing illustrious guests passing through the great archway into the courtyard beyond, the sound of music and voices raised in merriment spilling from within into the dark street where torch-bearers and coachmen stood chatting, waiting to be summoned by their masters. For a moment she seemed to have stepped back centuries in time to when the great house had been filled with life and laughter.

"Nowadays you find all sorts of little shops and restaurants in the Marais. Lots of Jewish people live here and there are small businesses tucked away as well, making everything you can imagine – goldsmiths, shoe-makers, book-binders – and all sorts of other skills and crafts."

Holly led Flo up a narrow alley until they came to a wooden door so time-worn that the heavy metal ring serving as a knocker had made a deep dent in its surface. It opened on creaking hinges to reveal a tiny elf of a woman. She must have been fifty or sixty years old, it was impossible to tell. Her hair was dyed bright red with henna and she was dressed in an assortment of colourful clothes which could at best be described as eclectic. A pair of gold spectacles hung on a chain round her neck. Holly embraced her fondly. "This is Leah." She introduced her to Flo and the two rather formally shook hands.

They entered what appeared to be a workroom with a large square table in the centre that was laden with bolts of cloth, some partly unwound. Leah pushed them roughly to one side and Holly opened the folder which she had brought with her. She spread her designs for the other woman to see. Immediately they began a lively conversation in rapid French.

Unable to follow, Flo looked around her. Along one side of the room there was a metal rack with grey, black and navy clothes on hangers. At first sight she took them to be men's suits, but when she approached closer, she saw that they were beautifully-tailored trouser suits for women. She opened one of the jackets, admiring the lightness of the fabric, the quality of the buttons, the exact stitching of the buttonholes, and the smooth silk of the lining. Then her eye fell on the neat white label with its three words printed in black. *Holly de Valmont*, she read.

Leah and Holly came over, deep in discussion. Flo saw her friend examine the garments one by one, turning them inside out to look at the seams, scrutinising every tiny detail. She looked more than satisfied, and when she slipped one of the jackets on she did not stand in front of the mirror but stretched her arms and bent backwards and forwards. Flo saw how the perfect cut made the fabric seem to flow with her movements.

An hour later they were sitting drinking Russian tea from a silver samovar which was bubbling in one corner of the room. In broken English Leah told them how she and her family had fled from their native St Petersburg after the October revolution in 1917 and, like many emigrants from Russia, had found refuge in Paris. Although her family had once been wealthy, Leah had then been obliged to learn a trade to support herself, and had become a seamstress.

"Leah is one of the best in the whole of Paris," Holly burst in warmly. "She could work for any of the great couture houses, but she won't."

Leah tipped the ash from her black Sobranie cigarette. "I do not want to work for the establishment." She had a deep husky voice from long years of smoking, and her English was heavily accented. "I want to help young designers, like Holly. One day her name will be known all over the fashion world and I will say, I, Leah Goldman, I work for her when she was only a leetle Engleesh girl in Paris and nobody know her!" They all laughed, but Leah's eyes were serious.

The afternoon was drawing to a close when Holly and Flo found themselves outside in the narrow street once more. Flo had so much to say, she did not know where to begin. Sensing her friend's need to talk, Holly stopped the car on their way home at Les Halles where they sat down in one of the cafés bordering the now empty market stalls.

"Holly," Flo began as soon as the waiter had placed their espressos in front of them, "why didn't you tell me you actually have your own label? It's fantastic."

"I haven't had it for very long. This is just the start. Arlette put me in contact with Leah – they've known each other for years. I'd never have found her on my own. She's wonderful. She has a team of women who work for her. Most of them are Russian Jews like she is, and they make up the garments."

"And how are you going to sell them?"

"I took some samples to various boutiques in the Marais

quarter and two of them agreed to include my clothes in their range. Everything I've given them so far has been snapped up at once and several customers have even given me commissions to copy the styles in other colours or materials."

Flo leant over the table and squeezed her hand. "I'm so happy for you. Are the clothes very expensive?"

"Well, they're not exactly cheap. The fabrics are top quality and Leah and her team don't work for nothing of course, and the shops take their cut as well. But I still want ordinary working women to be able to buy my clothes, perhaps not very often, more like an investment they can afford just now and again."

"That's great." Flo drained her little cup before looking earnestly across the table at her friend. "But Holly, you've got to think of yourself and Rose as well. It's a lot of work. Are you sure it's all going to pay off for you?"

Holly shrugged. "Even with my poor grasp of mathematics I can see there's only a tiny profit in it for me right now. But this is what I really want to do, and it's important to get my name established in the trade."

"But Rose and you have to live off something as well. You're going to have to start thinking like a businesswoman, not just like an artist, you know."

Holly sighed. "That's my biggest problem. Fortunately I have the Montefiori contract which pays the rent, but I still rely on the work I do for Arlette for the rest of my income. It's such a pity she's away in Deauville at the moment. I'd have loved you to meet her."

"I'd have liked that, too." Flo picked up the bill and signalled to the waiter. "What sort of work do you do for her?"

"Researching for articles for the magazine, copy-writing, a bit of editing – general dogs-bodying. Sometimes I have to stand in for her at photo shoots or various public relations functions. Officially I'm her part-time PA, but sometimes I think the job's her way of keeping me financially above water since Rose was born. She adores Rose . . . I don't know what I'd do without Arlette."

Flo paid the bill, but when the waiter had gone they stayed sitting, listening to the birds in the trees, the rush-hour traffic no more than a muffled roar in the distance.

"It's so beautiful here." Flo's eyes ran over the stone facades of the surrounding buildings glowing in the golden light of the summer evening. "I wish I didn't have to leave tomorrow."

"I'll miss you," Holly said simply. "So will Rose. Promise you'll come and see us again soon."

Flo's voice was stern as she rose to her feet. "It's your turn to come and visit me first!"

Holly said nothing, but in bed that night she lay awake for a long time, wondering when she would find the courage to go back . . .

NINETEEN

North Yorkshire, October 1963

. . . Holly once again glances anxiously at her watch. Ten to eight. Nervously she checks the table. Two places are set for dinner. She rearranges the paper napkins. Too soon to light the candles, best wait till she hears his car pulling up outside. She turns down the oven. Good that she decided to make a chicken casserole, at least it will stay warm without overcooking. Nick should have been here by now. This is so unlike him.

She peers out of the window for the twentieth time. It looks onto a narrow lane with terraced houses on either side, one of many terraces down by the docks in Middlesbrough, a grimy relict of what was once a booming industrial town. The neighbourhood is run-down, and there is a tension on the streets between the black and white communities that she can physically feel. She sees only three boys outside, in school uniform, kicking a football about in the failing light of the autumn evening. As she watches, a woman's voice calls and they reluctantly pick up their ball and disappear from view. A car passes by, its headlights dipped, but does not stop.

Where is he? Perhaps something has happened? An accident? He always drives so fast. She wanders aimlessly through her tiny flat, trying to distract herself. She plumps the cushions on the sofa that takes up most of the sitting-room, then smoothes the fresh linen on the bed they will share in the even smaller bedroom. She has furnished the first floor apartment with pieces taken from the farmhouse, but although they were her mother's best, they are not antique. Nor are they modern and elegant like the teak range in fashion at the moment. Just post-war utility furniture, very plain, scarred and scuffed with the marks of her childhood.

She has done her best to make the rooms cheerful and comfortable, sewing new curtains and covers with cheap fabric off the market and she feels at home here now. She will never forget her relief when the bank informed her that the sale of the farmhouse, after deduction of all the debts, would leave her a tiny sum, enough to live on during her one-year pre-diploma course in textile and fashion design at the local art college. The rent is low and she is used to living on a tight budget, supplementing it by giving French lessons to a girl from the local grammar school. The art course is good, her tutors are encouraging and she can see how her skills are developing, but it is only at the weekends that she really comes alive, when Nick drives up from London to see her. Not every weekend, but about twice a month, like now.

Tyres on the tarmac outside, an engine stopping, a car door slamming – she knows the signs. She rushes to the door and runs down the stairs to meet him.

"Oh Nick, where have you been? I've been so worried!"

"Hey, I'm here now." He has dropped his bag and is taking her in his arms, whirling her off her feet. They share a long kiss before going into her flat.

"I thought you must have had an accident. You're usually here by seven. What happened?"

"I had to drop a fellow off in Leeds on the way up. Couldn't really say no because he was paying for the petrol. These are for you." He zips open his bag and pulls out a box of chocolates tied with a green and gold ribbon.

"Thank you. They're lovely." Holly stares at the box. He has never brought her anything before. "We can share them as dessert when we've had our meal."

"Oh, I stopped and had a bite to eat in Leeds. I was starving." He glances at the table she has set. "Sorry, darling, I didn't realize you'd go to all this trouble, cooking dinner."

"It's alright. I should have thought you'd have eaten by now. It doesn't matter. We can have it tomorrow instead." As she switches off the oven, she feels his arms slide round her waist.

"I can think of something I'd far rather be doing than eating dinner." His lips are nibbling her ear, sending delicious thrills down her spine. "Let's take that bottle of wine with us and drink it somewhere a lot more comfortable . . ." He is leading her into the bedroom, his hands lifting her skirt, pressing her to his body. She feels his arousal.

"All these clothes are really unnecessary, you know." They are lying on the bed and he is opening the buttons of her shirt one by one. "And whoever invented these terrible tights? Very off-putting. Why don't you girls wear stockings with lovely suspenders any more? They were a lot nicer. Mmm, that's better." He bends his head and covers her breasts with tiny kisses that send shivers to the core of her being.

All the week's cares and worries melt away as they slowly make love, then, when he has aroused her desire to the point where she thinks she can stand his caresses no more, he enters her, pressing into her gently at first, then deeper and deeper, faster and faster until they climax as one.

Nick rolls onto his back, one hand over his brow. She loves the moment when he takes her in his arms afterwards and kisses the tip of her nose. Usually they fall asleep then, their arms and legs entwined, but this evening she is surprised because he wants to talk.

"Why don't you come back to London with me?"

"What? Now?" She thinks he is joking or that it is his way of starting to say how much he misses her, but he insists.

"This place is so damned far away. I don't see what keeps you here. I mean, this flat isn't exactly what you'd call fabulous, is it? London is full of art colleges. You can do a course there like you're doing here and we can be together every day. And you could move into my flat with me. I've got enough room."

She is both hurt and stunned, superficially hurt that he should criticize her home, but on a deeper level bewildered: this is the first time he has not supported her in all the difficult decisions she has had to make since her mother died.

"I thought we agreed that I should stay on here to take my

pre-dip course. It does exactly the subjects I want. You know I couldn't afford to live in London on the money I've got and I couldn't stay in your flat for free. We've been through this before." She is on the defensive, speaking carefully, rationally, trying not to show how his words have upset her.

"Yes, but I don't see the point any more. It takes up so much time driving backwards and forwards, not to mention the small fortune I'm spending on petrol."

She tries to see his view of things. At all costs she wants to avoid a quarrel. The weekend is so short, every hour so precious, why are they going on like this? She tries to keep her voice steady, not to let him see how wounded she is.

"Of course, Nick. It's so wonderful that you manage to make the time to come and see me and I'll go halves on the petrol with you if you like . . ."

He is swift to realize that he has gone too far. "I'm sorry, Holly, I didn't mean what I said just now. How could I be such a fool as to speak like that! Forgive me." The grey eyes are pleading with her. She longs for them to crinkle with laughter again.

"It's alright. You do so much for me. I know you didn't want to hurt me."

"How could I ever hurt you, my darling?" He kisses her lips tenderly. "It's just that I miss you so. I want to see you more often than a couple of weekends in a month."

"Maybe I'll get accepted for a diploma course at the London College of Fashion. My tutor agrees that I should definitely study fashion design rather than fine art. He says I should apply soon to get a place for next year. Wouldn't that be great? Then we'd be able to see each other all the time."

He seems grateful for the change of subject. "I know you'll love London. It's such an exciting place to be right now. The clubs there are really fantastic."

She has not realized before that he must go out during the week. Her own life is so centred on the weekends, it is hard to imagine him going out and having a good time without her.

"You must get to hear some great groups."

His eyes glow in the lamplight as he turns towards her, propping himself up on one elbow.

"There are some incredible ones around right now, like The Hollies, and The Kinks. Everyone in the clubs is raving about them."

"I still like The Beatles best."

"Don't you think John Lennon's brilliant?"

"Yes, but I'm a Paul McCartney fan really," she confesses. "I'd give anything to see them play live."

"I went to see them last week at the Hammersmith Palais."

"And?" Holly holds her breath expectantly. "What were they like?"

"Haven't a clue!" he replies cheerfully. "Worst concert I've ever been to. All the girls in the audience stood on their seats as soon as the curtain rose and screamed hysterically from beginning to end. I couldn't hear a single note!"

"What a pity," she says, thinking that she might have done exactly the same.

"But the best group I've ever heard are The Rolling Stones. They were on at the jazz club in Ealing. Absolutely fantastic! Some people say they're going to be bigger than The Beatles. What do you think?"

"I've never heard of them," Holly confesses. She sometimes feels that Nick has entered her quiet little world from another planet.

Her answer seems to please him. "Come here, my little country mouse." He takes her in his arms and holds her tight. Long after he has fallen asleep she lies there, listening to his steady breathing, feeling warm, safe and loved.

The next morning they sleep late and then make love again. When they get up at last, the weather is sunny and warm for October so they skip breakfast and take a flask of coffee and some rolls to the beach, where they find a spot that is sheltered from the cool north-easterly breeze. Holly has brought her sketchbook and draws Nick's portrait as he dozes in the sun. She sensually traces his long limbs and lithe figure with her pencil, and is trying to capture the relaxed expression on his sleeping face when he wakes with a start and sees her, pencil in hand.

"Can I have a look?"

"No, not till I've finished."

But his curiosity gets the better of him and he comes over to admire her work. "It's not for college, is it?"

She does not understand his question. "Of course not. We don't do portrait painting on my course. Why do you ask?"

"I just wondered." His answer is deliberately vague. She knows there is a reason for his question, something that he is hiding from her.

"Nick, is there any work *you* should be doing for your college course right now?"

He is pretending to look out to sea, not meeting her eyes. "Oh, there's an anatomy exam coming up on Tuesday, but it's nothing to worry about. It's nothing important. I'll get stuck in when I get back on Monday. Boring stuff, really."

"It may be boring but you've still got to learn it." The moment the words are out she wishes she had never spoken. She sounds like her former history teacher at school. Nick is looking at her like a recalcitrant schoolboy. She quickly adopts another line of approach.

She gets to her feet and puts an arm round his waist. They watch the waves breaking like froths of lace onto the sand. "Nick darling, I know how much medicine means to you. I'd feel awful if the days you spent with me meant that you couldn't give enough time to your work. It's so important that you qualify and do what you've set your heart on. If there's anything I can do to help . . ."

Another quarrel has been averted.

He grins ruefully and looks down into her face. "My sweet Holly. It's so much nicer being here with you instead of learning ghastly anatomy." He looks down and scuffs the sand with his bare feet like a little boy who has been caught doing mischief. "But my marks haven't been too good lately and I only just managed to scrape through my last exam. My tutor's been on at me that I've got to put more effort into learning the basics, otherwise I'm not going to get anywhere in my finals."

"He's probably right," Holly says softly. "Don't you think so?"

"I suppose so. It's just that I couldn't bear not seeing you this weekend."

"I'm so glad you came. Have you brought your books with you?"

"Lord no. They're all in London."

"Then let's go back to my place now. We can have the dinner I cooked for us yesterday and after that you can drive back tonight. That way you'll have all tomorrow and Monday for your revision and you can impress your tutor!"

He kisses her gently on the lips. "You're right of course. You always are. My darling Holly, what would I do without you?"

The sun has vanished behind a bank of grey cloud that is drawing in from the sea. They pack their belongings and head for home. After a dinner that is eaten quickly and without wine, Nick takes Holly's face between his hands.

"Goodbye, my darling. I'll try to come up again in two weeks' time. I love you." He kisses her. "I'll miss you."

"I love you and I'll miss you too." She tries to hold back the tears that are filling her eyes but they overflow and start to run down her cheeks. He kisses them away before he turns and closes the door of the flat behind him.

She does not go into the street to wave. Their affair is already the talk of the neighbourhood and she does not want to fuel any more gossip. She hears the roar of the engine as his car pulls away from the kerb, and then he is gone.

When she starts to clear the dishes from the table she finds the chocolates Nick brought her which they have not had time to open. They are handmade, from Harrods, exquisite and expensive. She shakes her head. Dear, sweet, impulsive, generous Nick! She puts them on the kitchen shelf where they will stay till his next visit. Then she pours the rest of the previous evening's wine into a glass and takes it into her little sitting-room, slips a shilling into the meter and turns on one bar of the electric fire.

Its glow seems to reflect the warmth of Nick's love for her. He is even prepared to risk failing his exams in order to see her. She remembers his words 'What would I do without you?'

The question is rather, what she would do without him.

TWENTY

Paris, June 1969

Flo stroked the box containing her wedding dress lovingly before putting it with her suitcase into the back of Holly's car. "Thanks so much for everything. I've had such a great time. It's all gone so quickly. And thank you most of all for this!"

"I'm so glad you came. It's been great having you here."

"Oh Holly, Paris is such a beautiful city, so romantic. Mike and I can't afford a honeymoon, but if we could, this would be where we'd come. I can't wait to tell him about all the places we've been to and the lovely food and wine we've had. I don't know how you manage to live here and stay so slim."

Flo's chatter continued until they reached the Gare du Nord where she was to take the boat train to London. Holly looked at the huge board overhead listing the immediate departures and her eyes followed the crowds of travellers laden with luggage scurrying onto the platforms. The train was already in and Holly helped her friend lift her bags inside. A station attendant slammed the carriage door. Holly waited until Flo had found her seat and pulled the window down so they could say their final goodbyes.

"I wish I was going with you."

The vehemence of her own words surprised her so much that she tried to turn them into a joke, adding, "Then I could be sure that you don't forget the dress when you get off." She had often teased her friend about an incident years ago when Flo had lost a dress she had just bought in York, leaving the bag in the train going home.

This time Flo was not deceived. She looked at Holly keenly.

"You've built up so much here, even your own business. There's so much going for you. Your life is here now, Holly. In

Paris. And you've got Rose as well, don't forget that."

"How could I?" Holly smiled, her heart melting as it always did at the thought of her little daughter, but when the guard had blown his whistle and the train snaked its way out of the station, she was left with a sense of loss. Rose was safe in Marie-Jo's care, and although she had work to do, she could not face the empty flat just yet. Arlette would be back at the office that morning after her short break, so on an impulse Holly decided to go in and see her there.

The editorial staff of *Mode et Beauté* were housed in a futuristic construction of concrete, glass and steel that, like many new buildings being erected in Paris, blended into its classical environment in a genial symbiosis of ancient and modern. Holly took the elevator up to the top floor. By the time she reached it, her spirits had lifted already.

"Holly, how lovely to see you!" Arlette rose from behind her desk to embrace her warmly. "How is my darling Rose?"

"She's an angel except at nights when she's cutting her back teeth. Then she's an absolute devil."

Arlette laughed and motioned her to take a seat.

"How was Deauville?"

She did not need Arlette's enthusiastic response to see that the days on the Normandy coast had done her good. A light tan flattered her faultless complexion and her eyes sparkled with health. Since her marriage to Maurice at Easter she had become calmer, and the little crease between her brows had disappeared. Her new-found happiness had dispelled the ever-present air of sadness that had haunted her since losing her first husband and her little daughter, although at certain times – on their birthdays, their name-days and the anniversary of their deaths – she kept to her room, emerging red-eyed when the day was over. Maurice respected her past in the knowledge that her future lay with him. As a wedding present he had bought her a villa in Deauville, which they used at weekends or for short holidays to escape from the summer heat and pressures of city life. A house unburdened with memories, it was a new beginning for both of them.

Arlette had to be brought up to date on Rose's development. After ten minutes of close questioning and correspondingly detailed answers on Holly's part, she opened a file on her desk and took out an embossed invitation card.

"I'm afraid I have to ask you to do me a favour again."

"It's never a favour, Arlette," Holly protested. "After all, you're paying me to be your assistant." She often wished that she could do more to justify the sum which appeared in her bank account each month.

Arlette handed her the card. "There's a public relations do at the Ritz this evening, a promotional event run by one of our biggest advertising clients, so someone from the magazine has to be there. I'm sorry it's such short notice, but it arrived while I was in Deauville. No one else from the office is free tonight, chérie, so if you could go there, I'd be so grateful. We can't afford to offend this client. Just put in an appearance, that'll be enough."

"Of course. I'd be delighted to go." Holly spoke with more enthusiasm than she was feeling. She was pleased to be able to help, but she had attended enough PR events to be less than excited at the prospect of the evening ahead as she was well aware of the stereotyped pattern for promotions like this. She blessed Marie-Jo who would babysit for her once again, but at the same time her conscience pricked her and she decided to make up for her absence by taking Rose to the playground in the park that afternoon.

It was almost nine when Holly arrived at the Ritz. On entering the room where the promotion was taking place, she found herself caught up in a crowd of professional party-goers, minor celebrities with little more in mind than seeing their pictures in the next edition of *Vogue* or *The Tatler*. They all seemed to be acquainted, probably from their attendance at hundreds of similar functions, and the air reverberated with effusive greetings and extravagant compliments. Some of their outfits could only be described as bizarre, but Holly did not feel out of place in her black mini dress, sheer black stockings and patent leather sling-backs. Although it was the prescribed uniform for such occasions, it was not one in which she could relax. She thought of Rose at home, asleep in her cot. As soon as she had done her duty for Arlette, she decided she would slip away at the first opportunity.

For the moment there was no chance of escape. She was forced to wait until the official presentation of *Désirée*, the fragrance being launched, had run its course. The inevitable speeches were held. Free samples were snatched up by eager hands. Women were liberally spraying themselves with the new perfume and cooing with delight.

Holly took refuge at the back of the crowd where she found herself standing next to a man whom she took to be in charge of the catering; he had been presiding over the uncorking of the champagne and directing waiters with trays of canapés on her arrival. She was surprised when he suddenly turned and addressed her.

"What do you think of the new scent?"

"Wonderful," she replied drily, "for any woman over sixty whose life revolves round bridge drives, cocktail parties and society luncheons."

"That's exactly what I tried to tell my father, but he wouldn't listen to me." Holly's introduction to Michel Galliard, junior head of the House of Galliard, perfume-makers in the south of France since the eighteenth century, was complete.

"Holly Barton," she said simply and held out her hand.

Perhaps it was the fact that she did not make any excuse or apologize for her words, which attracted him. He had asked for her opinion and she had given it. Her honesty and straightforwardness seemed to appeal to him. The hand holding hers was warm and strong and when she withdrew it, he seemed slow to release it. He must be about five or six years older than herself, she guessed, tall and athletically built, as if he played a lot of sport or spent much of his time working in the open air. He had deep blue eyes – unusual for a Frenchman – framed with long black lashes, and he looked in amusement into her own. His thick hair was dark brown, falling in unruly curls around his sun-tanned face.

"Are you in the retail trade?"

His second question was totally professional. For some ridiculous reason she felt disappointed. Of course he must be interested in finding out whether she was a prospective client for his company. After all, she told herself, this was not a party. It was for commercial reasons alone that his family had gone to considerable expense to run this event. She answered his question coolly, telling him which publication she represented and handing him Arlette's business card. As she did so, she tried to avoid looking up into those deep blue eyes again.

A man whom Holly recognized from a previous function as a buyer at Galeries Lafayette, Paris's most glamorous department store, was approaching, and with a brief "Merci" and a friendly nod in her direction Michel Galliard excused himself and turned to greet him. The two had clearly done business before as after perfunctory greetings they launched into a discussion of prices and percentages. Holly moved away. A wave of tiredness swept over her, so strong that she had to suppress a yawn. It had been a long day since she had driven Flo to the station that morning. Flo would be on the train from London to York now. All of a sudden Holly missed her company, the warmth of her friendship and her easy English chatter. The party going on around her was livening up now that the official part of the function was over. The champagne was taking its effect. People on all sides were eating, drinking, smoking, talking, laughing and shouting, but she did not feel in any way involved. She did not belong here. Suddenly she could not stand it any more. She had to get out. She pushed her way through the crowd, took the lift down to the reception hall and ran outside where she almost threw herself into a waiting cab.

At home she found Marie-Jo stretched out comfortably in front of the television. Holly was glad that she wanted to go back to her own flat rather than stay and chat as they often did. Alone at last, she kicked off her shoes, pulled off the black dress, and leaving everything lying on the floor wrapped herself in her dressing gown and went into the kitchen where she made some tea. Closing her hands round the mug she sat down next to the cot where Rose lay fast asleep, one arm cast wide, the other clutching a furry rabbit, her gift from Flo from which she refused to be parted. Her eyelids fluttered on her soft cheeks and her parted lips curled in a smile. Perhaps she was dreaming of the happy hours they had spent in the park together that afternoon.

Holly rose and went to her own room. The air was mild; the heat of summer could not be far away. She opened the window and looked out into the moonlit garden where night transformed the sights and sounds of day. A strange creature slipped across the shadowy lawn. A bird she did not recognize screeched in the blackness of the cherry tree. Familiar had become unfamiliar and known unknown. Despite the warmth she shivered as she got into bed.

She lay in the dark, thinking with distaste of the people who had been at the event that evening. They had all seemed so superficial, as if they lacked any real values, except perhaps Michel Galliard. There was no reason why he should be any different from the rest, yet there had been something in his eyes which made her think he was. Nor was there any reason she should even remember him, he was after all only a business contact, but she could recall every detail of their meeting. How odd it was he should have had that effect.

She drifted from thinking to dreaming and Rose's smile played on her lips as she slept.

The following Saturday was warm, even for June. Holly had promised to take Rose to visit Arlette in the afternoon.

"Let's have tea outside today." Arlette led the way through the open doors of the salon onto the balcony. Maurice had gone hunting for the weekend and Arlette, who abhorred the idea of killing, had stayed in Paris. On the balcony overlooking a shady inner courtyard filled with lime trees, a wrought-iron table was set for two. There was delicate Limoges china, antique cake forks on lace napkins, a silver dish of madeleines and a plate of miniature chocolate éclairs. For Rose there was a glass of fresh orange juice. In Arlette's circle, as Holly knew from experience, no accommodation was made for the presence of children at the table; it went without saying that they were expected to behave accordingly. Mindful of recent spills at home, she took her daughter onto her lap.

Arlette poured tea into cups so transparent she could see the pale golden liquid through the bone china. Holly lifted Rose's glass to her lips but the little girl was tired after missing her midday nap. She put a chubby thumb into her mouth, nestled against her mother and fell asleep, leaving Holly secretly relieved that she could enjoy her tea without any fear of mishap. She loved being in Arlette's home again. Although she had an open invitation to come there, it was not often they found the time to meet outside the office; both had full schedules and, while Holly spent the rest of her time caring for Rose, Arlette was caught up in a social life that had increased since her marriage.

"Maurice and I are always so busy, we never seem to have a minute to ourselves." Arlette might have been reading her thoughts. "So it's bliss to get away to Deauville at the weekends. When are you and Rose going to come and visit us there? Maurice was saying only yesterday how long it has been since he last saw you both. I want to show you the house, it's so beautiful, and the beach will be perfect for Rose. I can't wait for her to see the sea."

"We'd love to come." Holly popped one of the tiny éclairs into her mouth. "Mmm, these are delicious."

"I told Madame Tourbie that you were coming so she made them specially this morning." Holly remembered the motherly cook who had so often prepared tempting dishes for her when she had lived under Arlette's roof. Those days seemed so long ago. Could it really be that only two years had passed?

They chatted as they sipped their tea, enjoying the drowsy warmth of the tranquil afternoon. A slight breeze chased hazy clouds across the azure sky and rustled the silvery leaves of the trees in the courtyard below. When they had finished, Arlette called Marie to clear the table and led the way into her study. Rose was sleeping soundly and did not wake as Holly gently put her into her pushchair.

"Now let me have a look at your latest designs." Arlette looked on expectantly as Holly undid the folder she had brought with her. She took out her sketches for the Grazia spring collection.

"I've pretty well got everything finished now, but I would like your opinion before I send them off to the Montefioris."

Where Flo had enthused effusively, Arlette only made brief comments on her work, suggesting a belt for a coat, changing the hem of a skirt or moving the buttons on a jacket. Holly noted her opinions eagerly. She did not need praise to know that Arlette was impressed.

"And now, tell me about your own collection. How is it coming along?" Arlette swept the papers back into the folder. The Italian designs were important, but she knew that Holly's main interest lay in creating her own label. "How are you getting on with Leah and her team?"

Holly's eyes shone. "They are fantastic. Leah and I are really on the same wavelength. She has such an eye. She seems to know intuitively what I want. I hardly ever have to make any changes and the quality of the work they do is superb. All the clothes have been snapped up so far. The boutiques take as much as I can deliver."

"That's wonderful – for a start, but you know you've got to get the whole idea on a more professional footing if you want it to be a success in the long run, don't you?" Despite her approval, Arlette was looking anxious.

"Yes, I know." Holly sighed inwardly. She had heard all this from Flo already. "It's just that I'm not really cut out to be a businesswoman."

Arlette's voice took on a serious note. "In this trade that's just what you've got to be. Believe me, I've seen enough talented young designers, some of them brilliant, who've tried to go it alone without managing the commercial side properly. All they are left with in the end is a pile of debts. I don't want that to happen to you. What about taxes, for instance?" Her voice softened. "Perhaps it would be a good idea if you had a talk with Maurice when you come to Deauville? I'm sure he could give you some very useful advice on that score."

"Would he really? That would be great."

"Of course. He'd be delighted to." Arlette watched as Holly put the sketches back into her portfolio. "And now come with me. It's my turn. I have something to show you."

She led the way to her boudoir where they so often used to meet in the mornings to discuss the day's work. The room had been freshly decorated but was as pretty and feminine as ever. There was no sign of Maurice's presence; the spacious apartment obviously afforded him his own bedroom and dressing room. Arlette opened a wardrobe and pulled out a suitcase. She placed it on the bed and flung it open. "These are for Rose. I have been keeping them all this time, but I want her to have them now."

Holly stared down at the contents. Neatly folded between layers of white tissue paper there were children's clothes, a little girl's wardrobe that could only have belonged to Virginie.

"Oh Arlette, are you sure? These things must mean so much to you."

"They do, but they won't bring my darling back." Tears sprang into her eyes and her voice trembled as she spoke. "I've clung to my memories for so long, too long perhaps. It is time to let go. I have Maurice now, and I have you and Rose, so I want her to have them. These were Virginie's prettiest things. She looked so sweet in them."

She sat down on the bed and gently lifted the top garment, a dainty sun-dress in shell-pink gingham with smocking on the front. Holly examined the tiny stitches; it was exquisitely hand-made. Suddenly she saw her mother again, sewing by the kitchen fire far into the night.

"Rose can wear it on the beach when you bring her to Deauville," Arlette went on. She picked up a dress in emerald green velvet edged with silk with a sash to match. "And this one should fit her at Christmas. Look, it's exactly the same colour as her eyes."

Holly was overwhelmed. "These are lovely, absolutely beautiful. I could never afford anything as gorgeous." Although the clothes were far too fine for everyday use, they would be perfect for Rose's visits to Arlette and Maurice instead of her usual dungarees. "How can I thank you?"

"Just come and see us as often as you can."

Arlette closed the suitcase with a bang as if she wished to change the subject so painful to her. They returned to the study where Rose was still sleeping peacefully. Arlette went over to her desk and handed Holly a slip of paper. "When I was in the office yesterday there was a call from a man who wanted to get in touch with you. He said it was a personal matter. I didn't give him your number as I didn't know who he was and one never knows these days, but he left his name and number so you can ring him back if you like."

Holly looked at the note in her hand. It said 'Michel Galliard', followed by a Parisian telephone number.

"Do you know him?"

"Not really. He was at that promotion I went to at the Ritz on Thursday evening where they launched the perfume I told you about."

"You mean he is one of the Galliards of Grasse, the perfume-makers?" Arlette's brows arched in surprise.

"Yes, the son, I think. We only spoke briefly. I wonder what he wants."

Arlette smiled. "I should think that's obvious. He said it was personal so he must want to get to know you. Tell me," she said with almost girlish enthusiasm, curling up on the chesterfield with her legs tucked under her, "what is he like?"

Holly sat down beside her. "He seemed very nice, attractive as well, I suppose." It was the best she could do. She had forgotten his face and how could she describe the way those deep blue eyes had looked into her own?

"That sounds a bit vague to me, considering he's one of

France's fifty most eligible bachelors – we did a feature about them once. The perfumery is in Grasse, in Provence, the family lives on the Côte d'Azur and the son is in charge of their Paris office. He manages the commercial side of the business. This must be him!" Arlette reached out and squeezed her hand. "You know you should go out more. It's not natural for someone as young as you to work all the time and stay at home in the evenings. I know you've got Rose to look after, but there's Marie-Jo and if she can't babysit you can always bring Rose here if you want to go out. I really mean that," she added. "I think you should ring him right away. Promise me you will."

Holly smiled. "With an offer like that, how can I refuse?"

At her words Rose woke up, but hunger and the heat combined to make her fractious and Holly thought it wiser to end their visit.

On her return home she bathed and fed Rose, then put her to bed before she dialled the number. The deep male voice that answered the phone was instantly recognizable. His warm response when she said her name told her that he had been hoping she would call, yet he was unexpectedly brief.

"I'm sorry I had to break off our conversation at the Ritz. I looked to see where you were as soon as I was free but you'd gone by then. It'd be nice if we could talk some more. Would you have dinner with me tomorrow evening?"

Holly's mind reeled in surprise. "Er, tomorrow? You mean Sunday?" she stammered, realizing how gauche she must sound.

"Yes, there's a nice restaurant I'd like to take you to. I could pick you up at eight, if you like."

"Eight o'clock would be fine." She hoped she sounded more poised this time. After noting her address he said goodbye and rang off. Holly put down the receiver thoughtfully. Something told her that this invitation might lead to more than dinner. Was she prepared for that? More than four long years had passed since the day when she had wished her life would end. Could she face another relationship? Would she be able to cope?

TWENTY-ONE

A t seven the following evening, after Marie-Jo had taken Rose upstairs to her own flat, Holly stood in front of her wardrobe. She had no idea what sort of restaurant Michel would take her to and prayed that it would not be one of the gourmet temples she had visited with Julien. In the end she chose a white linen skirt with a matching belted jacket which she had made herself and which had since become one of the basics of her collection. Then, thinking that her outfit might be too casual if the restaurant should turn out to be very grand, she laid out a black silk top to go under it and high-heeled sandals. She decided to wear her hair loose, only light make-up and no jewellery other a pair of simple gold ear-rings that had belonged to her grandmother.

She showered and dressed slowly, savouring the luxury of taking her time. When she was ready, she looked in the mirror and was satisfied with the result. Nobody would have guessed that she had not been out on a date for over two years, that she had virtually no money and that she was the mother of a young child. Those were details, she decided, which Michel Galliard would definitely not need to know. Just for one evening she wanted to escape from all the burdens of her daily life and have a good time.

When the doorbell rang, she saw with a shock that she had spent a whole hour entirely on herself. She opened the front door. He was taller than she remembered and, if anything, even more attractive in casual clothes than in his business suit, but those dark blue eyes were just the same. She quickly stepped outside to greet him. There was no point in having him come in, letting him see the state of the flat with its jumble of assorted furniture and toys, playpen and pushchair.

He greeted her warmly with a light kiss on both cheeks and

followed her down the narrow garden path to where a taxi was waiting.

He held the door of the car open for her as she got inside. It was not until he sat down beside her that she realized that she had only spoken about a dozen words to this man before. In fact he was a total stranger to her and she to him, and yet her heart was beating with excitement. She felt like a teenager again. She told herself not to be ridiculous, but as the taxi pulled away from the kerb, a thrill of anticipation came over her at the thought of the evening ahead.

"There's a new little place in Saint-Germain. I haven't been there before but I've heard it's really good. We could try it out if you like?" His tone was courteous yet gentle. He seemed genuinely anxious to know whether she approved of his choice. Holly was reminded of dates with Julien on which he had always predetermined the venue, never asking her wishes. She pushed the unpleasant memory aside.

"That sounds lovely." She smiled and leant back in the cab. Already she was beginning to feel that she could relax in his company.

"Good. I booked a table, just in case." He smiled at her before leaning forward to give directions to the driver. They said little as the taxi wove its way through the evening traffic into the city centre.

Paris was at its most beautiful. The golden rays of the setting sun turned silver as they glittered on the Seine, the plane trees lining the boulevards were lush with rich green leaves and the pavement cafés a kaleidoscope of colour and movement. When they reached Saint-Germain, the student quarter near the Sorbonne university on the Left Bank, they stopped in front of a restaurant so small it could have been overlooked had it not been for the red-and-white checked cloths on the tables outside.

The proprietor greeted them cheerfully and led the way towards a table set for two. They sat down and a moment later he came over again to light the candle and take their order. There were no printed menus, the dishes being chalked on a board that was placed before them, and he proceeded to describe in detail the specialities of the day: fresh langoustines caught in Brittany only that morning, a fine pâté de foie laced with armagnac from his special supplier in Périgord, a superb turbot he had chosen himself at Les Halles, a succulent rôti de boeuf from Charolais cattle that had grazed on the richest pastures in Normandy. When Holly chose the crayfish and fillet of turbot, Michel announced that in that case he would have the pâté and the beef; after all, he laughed, it was the only way to be sure of not offending their host. When their order had been taken, two carafes of house wine appeared unsolicited, white for her and red for him. They raised their glasses.

"To this evening," he said simply.

She made no reply but smiled back into his eyes, midnight blue like dark still pools of water. There was a calm and quietness about him which appealed to her, but at the same time, he seemed vibrant with energy and life. When he discovered that she was not French, he at once switched into English. He spoke fluently with only a slight French accent – not because he had been a good pupil at school, he joked, but because he had spent two years at business school in London and had not yet had time to forget the language. The waiter brought the first course to their table. The food looked and smelt delicious.

"Tell me about yourself."

As they ate, she found herself talking about her daily life, working for Arlette at the publishers, designing the Grazia collection, and even her dream of having her own label. She did not try to make it sound glamorous as she might have been tempted to do with any other stranger. He listened intently, never interrupting, and then, not realizing that she was breaking her former resolution, she went on to speak of Rose, how sweet and funny she was, but also how hard it was to bring up a child alone.

"And Rose's father?" he asked softly.

"We are no longer in touch."

He looked understanding and sympathetic. "You'll make it," was all he said. She felt relieved that he did not try to give her tips or advice. She could not remember ever feeling so relaxed.

"Now it's your turn," she announced as the plates from the first course were cleared away.

He smiled. "Well, there's not a lot to tell. My family has owned land in Grasse for generations." When she broke in to confess that she had no clear idea where Grasse lay, he drew a little map on his paper napkin to show her. "Here, inland from the Riviera, in the Alpes-Maritimes. The climate, the slopes of the hills facing the sun, the soil and the water are all ideal for growing flowers, especially lavender, and are the basis for making perfume – which is what my family has been doing for over two hundred years."

Holly was fascinated. "Do you still use flowers today?"

"Of course." Her interest seemed to please him. "But we use other ingredients too, like patchouli, which is an oil from the leaves of a herb found in Asia. We even use animals, for example the musk deer for mochus or musk oil. To me, perfume-making is an art, not a science, and one that fascinates me. The other students at business school, they only wanted to market products – cars or cornflakes – they didn't care what it was as long as it would sell. But I don't think like that. My family's tradition means a lot to me."

He turned to other subjects and revealed that, despite his training in commerce, he had a love of art and music. Holly was delighted that he always asked her opinion on the topics they discussed. In many cases they discovered that they shared the same tastes, but she never had the feeling he was trying to instruct her or impose his views on her.

Suddenly Holly realized that all the other diners in the restaurant had left. Darkness had fallen and they were alone. More than three hours must have passed. Michel raised his hand to call for the bill, but instead the patron came over with a bottle of Calvados and three glasses which he filled at their table.

"I am happy to see you enjoy your evening so much," he said in his heavily accented English, clinking his glass against theirs. "That is what a good dinner is, not just great food but a great experience. I think you have had such a dinner tonight."

Holly took a sip of the amber liquid, its rich taste of apples caressing her palate like a delicious dessert, and as she swallowed she heard Michel say quietly, almost to himself, "C'est vrai, monsieur, you are right."

When the taxi stopped in front of her apartment, Michel escorted her to the door. His face was in shadow but she knew that those eyes were looking into hers. He bent his head and kissed her softly, no more than brushing his lips against hers. "Thank you for a wonderful evening." His voice was gentle and sincere.

She was tempted to invite him in. Somehow it did not seem to matter any more what the flat looked like inside, but before she could do so he spoke.

"I have to go. I have a long way to drive tonight."

She looked up at him, puzzled by his words, wondering whether she had heard correctly.

"I have to be in Grasse for a meeting with my father at eight in the morning. The last plane to Nice left at ten, so I missed it and I have to take the car instead."

"But . . ." she began, then paused. It was really none of her business what he chose to do.

"I know what you're thinking," he laughed. "Don't worry, I'm not going to drive myself there, I've had far too much wine for that. I'm taking one of our company cars, so it's the chauffeur who'll be doing the driving, but he's coming to pick me up at my apartment now. I'm sorry, I have to go."

"Good night, and thank you," she whispered. "Bonne route."

"Au revoir." He vanished into the night.

Holly closed the door of her flat slowly behind her, deep in thought. He had missed his plane so that he could spend an evening with her; the assumption was flattering. On the other hand, she wondered, how much actual hardship was there in having to sit in a luxury car all night and be driven by a chauffeur? Probably not a lot, she conceded wryly as she made her way to her bedroom, picking up toys and clothes on the way. Nevertheless she felt pleased with the way the evening had gone and could not help hoping, as she drifted into sleep, that more of the same might follow.

She was not to be disappointed. The phone rang the following morning while she was having breakfast in the kitchen with Rose.

"How are you today? I wanted to thank you for a beautiful evening." The warmth of his voice told her that it was not convention that had prompted him to phone.

"I'm fine, but I'm the one who should be saying thank you."

As in their previous telephone conversation, he came to the point immediately. He seemed to have no time for exchanging pleasantries. "I have to be here in Grasse till Friday, but I'll be back in Paris at the weekend. Can I see you again then?"

Her heart beat faster. She tried to steady her voice. "That would be nice."

"On Saturday?"

"Yes, I'm free on Saturday evening."

"No, I didn't mean in the evening, though that would be great as well. I meant during the day. Say from ten o'clock, if that's not too early for you."

"No," she stammered, "it's not too early, it's just that I can't . . ." How could she tell him that she could not possibly ask either Marie-Jo or Arlette to take Rose on a Saturday morning, perhaps even for a full day? He clearly had no idea that having a child to look after meant you could not just drop everything at the weekend and do whatever you wanted.

"Rose too, of course," his voice cut into her thoughts. "I wanted to have a day out with both of you. You told me so much about her, I'd like to meet her. If that's alright with you?"

"That would be lovely." She wondered whether her tone conveyed the happiness that swept through her.

"Great. I'll pick you both up at ten. I'll bring a picnic as well. You decide where you'd like to go. Au revoir." He rang off.

When Saturday came, Holly was relieved to see that the rain clouds which had hung over the city during the week had departed leaving a clear blue sky. It was going to be a perfect summer's day. She packed a bag with a sun-hat, nappies, food and drink for Rose, doubting very much whether the promised picnic would suit the tastes of a sixteen-month-old child. After dressing Rose in the pink sun-dress that Arlette had given her, she abandoned the jeans she had pulled on before breakfast in favour of a simple mini-dress in apple-green linen. As an afterthought she kicked off her sandals and put on a pair of espadrilles instead, placing comfort over fashion with the destination she had chosen in mind.

Michel was punctual. He embraced Holly, kissing her on both cheeks and complimenting her on her appearance, but greeted Rose only briefly as if he knew that she was shy with strangers and that he would have to win her confidence slowly. "Well, where are we off to?" he asked, as soon as they were seated inside the dark-green Alfa Romeo convertible with the bags and pushchair stowed in the boot.

"I'd love to go to Versailles," Holly suggested tentatively. "I've never been there before." She had been deliberating all week where they should go. The magnificent royal palace lay outside the city and ever since her schooldays when she had read the history of Louis XIV, the Sun King, she had longed to see it. It seemed the ideal place for an outing on such a beautiful midsummer day.

Michel seemed to think so too. "Wonderful," he announced, revving the engine as they drove down the quiet street. "I haven't been there for years. I think that's a brilliant idea."

Holly was relieved. At once she began to relax as she found it so easy to do in his company. The hood of the car was down and while they skirted the city before turning south, the noise of the traffic made conversation difficult. Michel turned the radio on. A medley of French and English pop music filled the air – hits by The Hollies, The Kinks and The Moody Blues interspersed with Johnny Hallyday, Françoise Hardy and Sylvie Vartan – songs of summer, songs of love, that made her cares fly away as fast as the wind that whipped the scarf holding back her long dark hair.

After parking the car, they strolled along the broad sun-lit terrace beneath the impressive façade of the great palace that overlooked bubbling fountains, sculpted gardens and landscaped paths. As they walked, Michel told her how Versailles had been built to house Europe's most powerful monarch and a court of thousands. "Louis XIV was known as Le Roi Soleil, the Sun King, because he saw himself, and France, as the centre of the universe, and he wanted this palace to reflect that grandeur so that everyone, especially the kings of Spain and England, would recognize his power. He was clever too, because he drew all the nobility here, like planets in orbit round the sun, and by doing that he had them all under his control and made sure that none of them questioned his authority by causing trouble elsewhere. Instead they neglected their estates at home and spent all their fortunes on trying to outshine one another at court!" He paused and pointed to the classical statues, clipped box hedges and stately cypresses in symmetry, lining the gravelled path they had taken. "Look how precise and orderly everything is, how controlled."

"There aren't any colours, any flower beds or gardens like we have in England," Holly noted.

"That's right. He wanted it to be a stage for the courtiers to show off their magnificent clothes. Nothing was allowed to detract from the elaborate fashions of the period. And of course the men were just as gorgeously and expensively dressed as the women, and just as vain!"

"Maybe they are today, too," Holly laughed. "Except that they find different ways to express it."

"I expect you're right," he grinned, "otherwise there wouldn't be so many expensive cars around! Let's have our picnic before we go inside the house."

They found a shady spot under a chestnut tree and Michel

spread out a rug before unpacking a range of delicacies that was far from the bread and cheese which Holly had expected. He lifted Rose out of her pushchair and sat her between them. An elderly couple passing by smiled and nodded in their direction; they must look like a young family on a weekend outing, Holly thought. She unscrewed a jar of apple purée for Rose but Michel took it from her and began to spoon the soft fruit into the little girl's mouth. Rose gurgled with delight, her green eyes never leaving his face. She waved her arms with excitement, knocking his hand holding the spoon so that its contents landed on his beige cotton slacks, but he just laughed and wiped the spot clean with a napkin.

When they had finished, they made their way slowly towards the palace. The afternoon sun was beating down, it was the hottest day of the summer so far and Holly was glad when they paid their entrance fee and entered the cool building. Rose's eyes closed, her curly head lolled to one side and she fell asleep in her pushchair as they walked. The empty shell of stone, once filled with pomp and grandeur, echoed to the hollow ring of their footsteps as they passed through its chambers.

Afterwards Michel took her to see Queen Marie-Antoinette's idyllic hamlet hidden in the grounds. As they walked he told her how, two hundred years ago, Louis XVI's tragic queen and her ladies had relieved the boredom of courtly life by dressing up and pretending to live there as shepherdesses, little knowing that they were soon to mount the steps to the guillotine. When they came to the fairytale village in its picture-book setting, Holly seemed to hear the tinkling sound of laughter echoing down through the centuries. She found herself wondering whether she might catch a stray glimpse of a billowing gown disappearing behind the trees or a powdered head peeping through one of the casement windows of the mill.

On their return to the car, Rose woke as they lifted her out of her pushchair and began to cry. Holly sat in the back with her, making conversation with Michel almost impossible. Despite her efforts, Rose refused to be calmed. Her sleep in the heat had not refreshed her and her face was flushed. "I'm sorry," Holly apologised, "I'll just have to bath and feed her and put her to bed as soon as we get home."

Michel smiled at her in the mirror. "Of course. It's been a long day. She's been very good." He said no more. When he pulled up in front of her flat, Holly got out with Rose on her arm and he carried her baggage to the door. "I'll phone," he said, bending to kiss her. A thrill went through her at the touch of his lips but a second later he had turned and gone.

She went wearily inside. Rose's crying had risen to a steady wail that reverberated through her head. "It isn't fair," she thought bitterly. "It's Saturday night and here I am, stuck at home with a screaming child." Moments like this were rare, she knew, but when they came they were hard to bear. The idea of ending the day dining in a lovely restaurant with Michel was a much more attractive thought!

She spoke soothingly to Rose, and by some minor miracle the little girl was suddenly quiet. A smile appeared on her face like a rainbow after a storm. Holly hugged her close. Whatever happened, she had her daughter to love. But deep within her a voice was asking whether that would be enough.

July was packed with deadlines and appointments. Holly no longer felt guilty about not doing enough work for Arlette; the holiday season had begun and she had to stand in for various members of staff on the magazine. Without Marie-Jo's help she did not know how she would have coped.

After hectic hours in the office she looked forward to the evenings when Michel asked her to dine with him in one of the many little bistros in Saint-Germain. He introduced her to the hearty country dishes for which France was famous: coq au vin from Burgundy, cassoulet from the Auvergne, bouillabaisse from Marseilles, choucroute from Alsace, all equally delicious. At weekends they went on outings with Rose: a boat trip along the Canal St Martin, a ride to the top of the Eiffel Tower or, on one rainy afternoon, a long walk through the Père Lachaise cemetery where the dripping branches of trees weeping over gothic tombstones exuded a morbid charm that Holly found enchanting.

Wherever they went, Holly was amazed how easy it was to talk to Michel, how much their views and feelings coincided despite their different backgrounds. He loved his country's culture, but he never tried to educate her. His tastes were simple. Where Julien had taken her to the Comédie Française, Michel took her to a performance of *Guignol*, the French version of Punch and Judy, in a tiny puppet theatre tucked away in the Marais; where Julien had taken her to the opera, Michel took her to hear Joan Baez at an open-air folk festival; where Julien had taken her to the Louvre, Michel took her to the Jeu de Paume gallery where she fell in love with the Renoirs at first sight.

Once they climbed up the cobbled streets to Montmartre to watch the artists painting, returning through Pigalle where garish-coloured lights lured tourists into spending their hard-earned dollars and pounds in the Lido and Moulin Rouge. Sometimes they just sat in one of the open-air cafés on the Boulevard St Michel, watching the never-ceasing spectacle of passers-by: purposeful businessmen with briefcases on their way home, busy housewives with baskets of vegetables and baguettes hurrying to cook their family's evening meal, students from the Sorbonne with books stuffed into their pockets, and lovers, always lovers, their heads bent close together, arms entwined.

"Arlette has invited Rose and me to visit her in Deauville this weekend."

They had met in a café after work. An evening breeze was beginning to cool the heat of the day. Holly stirred her coffee before she spoke again. "You are invited as well."

"Please tell her I'd be delighted to come." As ever his reply was brief.

"She'd like us to arrive on Saturday morning and stay till after lunch on Sunday if we can."

"Fine. In that case I'll pick you and Rose up on Saturday at nine thirty."

"Thank you."

She did not say more. The hours, even entire days she had spent in his company during the weeks they had known each other had always ended when he escorted her home. They had kissed, but never more than that. She had not once seen his flat, nor had he been in hers.

There was a barrier which stood between them. She could not prevent it. It was there, and she knew that he was aware of it too.

TWENTY-TWO

Deauville, July 1969

Though she had heard much from Arlette about her house on the Normandy coast, Holly was unprepared for the sight that met her eyes on their arrival. The stately double-fronted mansion overlooking the sea was imposing yet in many ways a family home, a house of nooks and crannies with red gabled roofs and tiny mansard windows, wooden verandas and shutters weathered by the sea air. From a garden cultivated in the English fashion, a flight of stone steps led down to a sandy beach. Arlette was at the door to greet them as their car pulled up in the drive.

"How lovely to see you all. Bienvenus à Deauville. Rose my darling, you've grown, come in and see what I've got for you." She took the little girl into her arms before turning to embrace Holly and stretch out one hand to greet Michel. He bent and kissed the air over her fingertips.

"Thank you for your kind invitation, Comtesse."

"Oh là là! Call me Arlette, please. And I may call you Michel?"

Holly was amazed. Although Arlette retained the polite, 'vous' form of address, she had opted to use first names with Michel. Such informality was unheard of in the echelons of French society to which they both belonged. Along with her conventions, Arlette had also abandoned her usual formal style of dress. It was the first time Holly had ever seen her wearing trousers, albeit beautifully cut slacks in navy-blue linen – Holly thought she recognized the hand of Saint-Laurent – but trousers nonetheless. A striped Breton-style top and a red chiffon scarf at her throat completed her maritime look. Leaving Henri to deal with their luggage, she led them inside.

The interior of the house was as welcoming as the exterior.

Passing through a hall where a magnificent vase on a round oak table held an exquisite arrangement of summer flowers, they entered the spacious lounge. Sofas with loose covers in shades of cream and gold gave the room a warmth which it would hold even when the sea that sparkled blue beyond the tall windows was shrouded in grey mists and rain. A radiogram with a sizeable record collection stacked beside it, a large television set, a cocktail cabinet and several coffee tables littered with magazines and books suggested winter evenings spent before the open fire. The atmosphere was one of leisure and comfort.

"Would you like a drink?" Arlette inquired. "You must be thirsty after your long drive." They passed through open doors onto the terrace. Under a green-and-white-striped awning, teak chairs with plump green cushions were grouped round a table bearing a huge bowl of peaches.

"Thank you, Frieda." Arlette nodded towards a grey-haired woman who placed a tray of glasses and a tall jug in front of them. "Frieda is our housekeeper here at Beau Rivage. She is from Bavaria. Her apple juice is more refreshing than the finest champagne, and her Kirschtorte . . . ," Arlette rolled her eyes, "is the most heavenly gâteau I have ever tasted, as you will judge for yourselves at dinner."

They had barely raised their glasses when Arlette was on her feet again. "Excuse us, please. Rose and I have to do some exploring on the beach. When you are ready, Frieda will show you to your rooms. Please make yourselves at home. Lunch will be here on the terrace at one o'clock."

Michel rose to his feet but she had already turned to leave, hand in hand with Rose. They watched as the two made their way through the garden and down to the beach.

"She loves Rose so much and thoroughly spoils her."

Michel reached over to take Holly's hand. "Let her. If it gives her comfort . . . " He said no more, smiling to see Rose stop and bend down to grasp a handful of sand, letting it run through her fingers in wonderment.

When they followed Frieda upstairs, Holly was not

surprised to see that Arlette, discreet as ever, had given them separate but adjoining rooms. Her luggage was waiting for her, the bed was made up with crisp white linen and there was a cot for Rose. As she unpacked she could hear Michel moving around next door and when she stepped onto her balcony, she found him standing on his, looking out to sea. They were so close they could have touched.

She breathed in deeply, drawing the salty air into her lungs, and when she exhaled it was as if she were expelling all the cares and worries of her daily life. She closed her eyes, letting the slight wind off the sea ruffle her hair. When she opened them again, Rose and Arlette were just tiny specks at the water's edge.

"Look how far the tide is out. I can hardly see them."

He laughed. "Somehow I don't think you'll be seeing very much of your daughter this weekend!"

After lunch they all walked along the sea shore, Michel carrying Rose on his shoulders, and by their return, she was almost falling asleep. Holly fed and bathed her before her eyes closed the moment she lay in her cot.

Holly showered and changed into a white dress of transparent cotton voile underlaid with silk. She did not know whether it was the day's sun or the anticipation of the evening ahead which brought a glow to her cheeks. Her steps were light as she descended the oak staircase for aperitifs in the lounge.

Holly paused before she entered. She could already hear Arlette and Michel deep in conversation. Was it simply that they belonged to the same social class that they possessed this innate ability to talk effortlessly on all topics, even with strangers, always maintaining the right balance between the superficial and the deep, the personal and the impersonal, the light-hearted and the serious? Did it come naturally along with wealth and ancestry? Even now, after living in France for so long, she sometimes wondered. And was it the knowledge of her father's genealogy that gave her the feeling that she too belonged in this world? She did not think so. Even if she had really been born a poor hill farmer's daughter, she knew that they would have accepted her with the same grace and kindness; it would have made no difference.

As if in response to her thoughts, Arlette and Michel broke off their conversation on seeing her and greeted her with open arms. Arlette's holiday wardrobe was in evidence once more; her evening black had been replaced by a simple shift in burgundy satin, a colour Holly had never seen her wear before but which suited her admirably.

"Maurice sends his apologies, ma chère. He has arrived late from the city and is changing." She had scarcely finished speaking before her husband entered the room. Accustomed to seeing him in a dark suit or dinner jacket, Holly wondered whether it was the navy blazer and grey slacks which made him look ten years younger or the happiness and well-being which radiated from him as he bent to kiss his wife.

"Holly, my dear, how lovely to see you again." He embraced her warmly and turned to shake Michel's hand. "Welcome to Beau Rivage."

As they sipped their drinks, Maurice told them more about the history of the house. The product of a bygone age, it had been built in the nineteenth century for the director of the Paris Opera House at a time when the Parisian upper classes were accustomed to holiday on the Normandy coast to escape the summer heat of the city. The Côte d'Azur had been a strictly winter playground then; no self-respecting aristocrat would have dreamt of exposing his wife's and his daughters' complexions to the dangers of the Mediterranean sun.

Holly listened, fascinated. "So the house was only used during the summer months?"

"That's right. The servants would be sent ahead from Paris to open it up and air the rooms before the family arrived for their vacation. The children would play on the beach, supervised by their nanny and governess; the parents would attend the races and the other social events that constituted the season here. Then, after seven or eight weeks, the dust covers would be brought out again and everyone would head back to the city. In a way they were not much different from us." He smiled at Arlette. "Except that we only manage to come here for a couple of days, not months."

"Yes, mon cher," his wife corrected him gently, "but at least we try to come the whole year round, not only in summer. I love the sea in winter."

"So do I." Holly had meant to go on but suddenly fell silent as a memory rose in her mind. A windswept beach, breakers crashing and the cries of sea gulls overhead, a pair of grey eyes that looked lovingly into her own, two arms that held her tightly. She was aware that Michel was watching her and took a sip of her martini to avoid meeting his gaze.

"Il est servi, madame." It was Frieda in the doorway. Arlette led the way into a panelled dining room where a table had been set for four. Compared to the dinners served in her Parisian apartment, the setting and food were simple, but superb nevertheless. An entrée of dressed crab, freshly caught, was followed by tender escalopes of veal with new potatoes and a green salad. After a locally-made Camembert cheese, Frieda's pièce de résistance, the famed cherry torte, arrived to a chorus of praise from all sides. Maurice served the wines, all white, himself: a light Chablis, then a full-bodied Alsatian Gewürztraminer to accompany the meat and cheese courses, and a vintage champagne with the gâteau.

Their conversation was swift and punctuated with laughter. Holly felt happy, knowing she was among friends. Michel too seemed completely at ease, amusing them with tales of his life as a Provençal in Paris.

When they reached the dessert, Maurice turned to Holly.

"And now, ma chère, I have been hearing many good things from my wife about your talents. How are your plans progressing?"

Holly told him briefly about her assignment for the Montefioris and her designs under her own label, taking care to mention her gratitude to Arlette for providing her with the regular salary which made all her designing possible. Maurice listened closely, watching her astutely. When she had finished, he crumpled his napkin and placed it beside his plate before replying. "Courage, ma petite."

Holly looked at him in surprise. The word meant the same in English as it did in French.

"What you need is courage. You say the owners of these boutiques are taking up the garments you produce with this – how is she called – Leah?"

"Yes," Holly replied, wondering where courage came into all this. "The problem is that the boutiques take so much of my profits that I don't make enough money on the clothes to support myself and Rose. That's why –" She paused and drew a deep breath. She was voicing her idea for the first time. "That's why I think I should produce more. There's certainly more demand for my clothes out there."

She stopped abruptly. Maurice was shaking his head.

"I have not seen these garments, but I gather from my wife that it is their quality, together with the design, that makes them so special. My dear, if you go into mass production, so to speak, you will dilute that quality and you will dilute the attraction of the label, too. No woman wants to be seen in a suit that another woman in her office is wearing. For that she can buy from La Redoute!"

It hurt to hear her work compared with the popular mail order firm. "But what can I do, apart from produce more?"

"Sell them yourself! That is the answer! Cut out all those boutiques who are taking all your profits. What are they doing for their money? They just hang your clothes on a rail! You can do that and you can do it better, because you have designed those clothes with your customers in mind. You know what suits them better than anyone else does."

Holly's thoughts were racing. "But to do that I'd need my own shop."

"That is true."

"But I haven't any retailing experience. I wouldn't know where to start."

"There are others who have!" It was Michel speaking, his eyes shining with excitement. "The whole operation just has to be organized properly."

"Exactly." Arlette joined in. "That's the future. A shop that sells only one brand so that the women who want those goods know exactly where to go. And of course it must be in a top location, in keeping with the quality of the products."

"Just a minute." Holly felt that the situation was getting beyond her control. "This is something I'll have to think about. And anyway," she looked levelly at her companions, "where would I get the money to do it? That sort of venture would need capital, real money. I could never afford it."

"That's where I come in." Maurice drained his champagne glass. "If you can find a location and draw up a viable business plan, I'd back you."

Holly could hardly believe her ears. "I could never accept that, Maurice. What if the shop weren't a success? I could never pay you back. I can't let you take such a risk."

"Whenever I invest I take risks, though needless to say I check my ground very carefully before I do. And now," he rose to his feet, "let us adjourn our little business meeting. I believe that Frieda has coffee for us in the lounge and I want to offer Michel some of my best port. But remember, my dear Holly, sometimes a little courage goes a long way."

The sea air had tired them all and it was just after eleven when Arlette and Maurice retired. Holly and Michel went upstairs together. Outside her room he bent to kiss her as he always did when the hours they had spent together came to an end, but this time it was different. Was it their new environment that freed them from the roles they had played until now? Holly did not care. She only knew that she wanted to stay in his arms and feel his lips on hers. She looked up and saw the longing in his deep-blue eyes.

"There's Rose," she whispered.

He nodded, understanding her unspoken desire, and led her to his own room where he did not switch on the light but pushed back the shutters. A full moon hung suspended over the swelling sea. He turned to face her, his body outlined in its pale shafts of light. She saw only his tall figure, his athletic build and the curly hair surrounding a face that was in darkness, but when he held out his arms she did not need to read his expression.

He held her tightly, caressing her through the flimsy fabric of her dress, kissing her face, her neck, her hair. For a moment he stopped and looked down into her eyes. "Holly darling, are you sure of this?"

"Yes," she whispered, and as if her words were not answer enough she pulled him towards her again. In response she felt his hands move to the fastenings of her clothes and they fell away one by one. Between kisses he pulled off his own garments and, when he stood naked in front of her, she felt so weak that it was a relief when he swept her into his arms and laid her gently on the bed.

His lips explored her body, touching her, tasting her, discovering her with all his senses. She wanted to return his caresses, but when she saw what delight her pleasure gave him, she relaxed and gave herself up to the enjoyment and, as she did so, her excitement seemed to arouse him further.

"We must be careful, my darling," he breathed in her ear. "We can't take any risks."

"It's alright," she whispered. "Nothing can happen." Silently she blessed Flo for her advice about the pill. She felt the weight of his body on hers, but then, suddenly, she was reliving all the agony of the rape, and panic seized her.

"It won't hurt this time." He held her tightly in his arms until the moment had passed.

Afterwards he lay beside her, tracing the outline of her lips with his finger in the moonlight. She looked into his eyes, as soft as velvet and as dark as the night. "You knew?"

He nodded. "Yes, I knew. I've known since our first date that something was there. I don't know why or how it happened, but I know that Rose's father hurt you badly. Perhaps even more badly than you realize. I was worried. Worried that it might stand in the way of my love for you."

"You love me?"

"Je t'adore." He took her in his arms again.

As the first rays of dawn began to touch the horizon they made love once more, slowly and deliberately, and this time there was no moment of panic but only ecstasy for both of them. Afterwards they lay together at peace and drifted into sleep, their bodies moulded as one.

Holly awoke early to a perfect day. The cool breeze had dropped. A sprinkling of rain had fallen in the night and from the garden below the green freshness of the trees mingled with the sweet scent of the roses that bordered the terrace. Holly picked up her clothes and slipped back to her own room. Rose was still sleeping so she pulled on her shorts and a shirt and crept barefoot downstairs.

No one was awake. All was quiet as she passed through the lounge, crossed the terrace and went down the garden to the beach. The tide was in. The air was so still that the vast expanse of sea barely moved. Only tiny waves lapped at her feet. She climbed onto a large rock at the water's edge, drew her knees up to her chin and sat staring into the distance.

She thought of Michel, of the night they had spent together, how happy she had felt in his arms. He had told her he loved her. She knew his feelings were deep and genuine, yet she was troubled. She had not responded. She had not told him that she loved him and, tender as he was, he had not pressed her to do so.

Did she love him? She loved so many things about him: his kindness and thoughtfulness, his affection for Rose, the way his eyes lit up when he talked and shone with understanding when he listened, the tastes and interests they shared, his looks, his smell, the touch of his body against hers. Was loving things about someone the same as loving that person? Surely love was more than that? She had loved once. She had given herself completely to Nick – body, heart and soul. Why could she not make that commitment again? She watched the swell of the sea as if the incoming tide would bring her the answer.

From behind, two arms suddenly encircled her and held her close. "What are you doing here perched on a rock, my little mermaid?"

"Wondering whether I should dive into the sea and swim away!" Holly laughed in his embrace, at the same time realizing that there was more truth in her words than there should have been.

"Don't you dare! I know two people who'd object. One is me, and the other's standing up in her cot, about to shout the house down if she doesn't get her breakfast."

"Rose!"

The spell that had turned her from mother into lover was broken. She scrambled to her feet and they raced each other back to the house.

Breakfast awaited her on the terrace when she came downstairs with Rose. "Alla! Alla!" The little girl stretched out her arms towards Arlette, her beloved Alla. The affection was mutual. Arlette glowed with pleasure and the high chair was placed next to her so that she could give Rose her breakfast.

"What's everyone planning on doing this morning? There are no rules here. Just please yourselves." Maurice was pouring coffee and handing round brioches and croissants with an unaccustomed air of domesticity. The once-confirmed bachelor seemed to be enjoying his household tasks.

"Well, we're going for a walk on the beach. We want to watch the tide go out and build a sandcastle, don't we, Rose?"

Rose, her mouth full of pain au chocolat, turned a beaming face towards Arlette and squealed with delight, her green eyes open wide.

"That means yes," Holly interpreted. "And if no one minds, I'd like to lie in one of those sun-chairs and do absolutely nothing."

"I'll join you."

At Michel's words, Holly glimpsed a smile flicker across

Arlette's face. Had she guessed the happenings of the night before?

"And I," Maurice announced, "will be in the garden checking what our gardener has been up to this past week. See you all at lunchtime, then. Let's say here on the terrace at one for aperitifs?"

The morning passed quickly. Holly lay in the sun, conscious of Michel's presence beside her, but the warmth soon made her drowsy and she fell asleep. At twelve she was awoken by Arlette and Rose returning from the beach with a bucket of shells to show her. Rose was tired but happy and let herself be put to bed for her midday nap.

Holly joined the others for lunch outside. A light meal was served, and after relating Rose's exploits on the beach, Arlette turned to the subject of holidays.

"Maurice and I will be here for three whole weeks in August." She leant across the table and squeezed her husband's hand. "It will be bliss to escape from Paris in the heat and stay for longer than two days at a time."

"I wish I could get away," Holly sighed, remembering how stifling the French capital was at the height of summer.

"Then join us, my dear. Rose would love it too."

"I've got a different idea – if you don't mind, Arlette?" Michel broke in with a courteous nod towards his hostess. "I'd like to invite Holly to meet my parents and see how we Galliards live down on the Côte d'Azur." He turned to face Holly. "Would you come?"

"That would be wonderful, but I'm not sure I can get away. What about the office, Arlette? Won't you need me during the holiday season? And what about my work with Leah? I can't just drop everything and go."

"Ma chère, it could be difficult for you to take three weeks, but one week should be no problem. And as for your business, you know that in August Paris is for the tourists only! All the Parisians who can afford it will have fled the city. There will be no one wanting to try clothes on in thirty degrees of heat! And

Leah works so hard, she deserves a break too."

"But what about Rose?" She knew it would be better not to take Rose to stay with strangers.

"Rose can stay with us!" Arlette was almost begging her. "You needn't worry, we can look after her. She'll have a wonderful time here and perhaps by the time she leaves she'll be able to speak quelques mots de français!"

Holly looked round at the circle of expectant faces. She knew Rose would be safe and happy in Arlette's care. She herself desperately needed a holiday and she had always longed to visit the Côte d'Azur. Perhaps the colours and light of the Riviera would provide inspiration for her work. Most of all she longed to spend more time with Michel. If she met his family and got to know him better, surely it would help to sort out her feelings for him.

"Well?" Michel's voice was anxious, his eyes pleading.

She smiled. "I think it's a marvellous idea."

TWENTY-THREE

Côte d'Azur, August 1969

Holly gazed over the sparkling waters of the pool to the magnificent white villa beyond, its windows shuttered against the midday sun. They had landed at Nice airport late the previous evening and arrived at La Mouette after midnight. It was only now that she was able to see the beauty of Michel's family home.

Her eyes dwelt on the tiered terraces of cool marble and the landscaped gardens of the estate, perched high on the Corniche above Cannes, commanding uninterrupted views of the Mediterranean. The deep azure of the sea and sky merged so perfectly that only the dots of the cruisers and yachts picking their way along the coast to Monte Carlo or Nice showed where the water ended and heaven began.

Michel rose from the sun-bed beside her. His towelling bathrobe fell away to reveal a tanned, athletic body in black swimming trunks. He stepped onto the diving board and the sun caught the muscles of his back, that tapered from broad shoulders to narrow hips. He raised his arms above his head and executed a perfect dive into the pool, barely causing a ripple. Holly watched admiringly, envying his obvious enjoyment as he swam powerfully in the cool depths, but felt far too indolent to join him. He surfaced in front of her and a thousand droplets glittered on his bare skin and in his dark hair. His eyes shone, vying with the intense blue of the water.

"Come on in. It's fantastic." When she shook her head in drowsy refusal, he heaved himself out with one effortless flowing movement to sit on the terracotta tiles beside the sun-bed where she lay. Holly murmured sleepy appreciation as she felt his hand gently rubbing her shoulders with sun oil. With slow, circling motions he massaged her body, moving from the nape of her neck to the small of her back. Acutely conscious of his fingers sliding sensuously over her skin, she pillowed her face on her forearms. She was blissfully happy. She was on the Riviera! She could hardly believe it. La Mouette was a far grander residence than she had imagined and she was looking forward to meeting Michel's parents that evening.

When she did so, she was disappointed to see that they were to be part of a large dinner party. She had hoped that his parents might use the occasion as an opportunity to get to know her better, but soon realized that this was not his mother's intention. In fact twelve sat down to dinner on the terrace overlooking the sea, her hosts presiding over their guests in a manner not dissimilar to that of Prince Rainier and his Hollywood princess holding court in their fairytale palace just a few kilometres along the coast.

At the head of the table François Galliard, Michel's father, was every English person's idea of a typical Frenchman. Short and wiry with black hair and eyes that twinkled with Gallic charm, he bent over Holly's hand before raising it to his lips.

"Mademoiselle, je suis enchanté."

His wife, an Austrian baroness by birth, seemed distinctly less enchanted. A statuesque blonde, almost a head taller than her husband, she kept a cool reserve. It was obvious where Michel had inherited his height and good looks, but while his blue eyes sparkled with gaiety and affection when turned in her direction, those of the baroness remained cold, and her chiselled features impassive. Holly sensed her anxiety regarding a liaison between her only son and this upstart of an English girl with an illegitimate child.

She had been placed opposite Michel and could feel his eyes approving her as she took her seat. The cream silk trouser suit was one of her own designs and superbly fitted the occasion – more so, she thought, than the stiff embroidered eveningwear of the other women present. Only the baroness, whose white chiffon tunic and loose palazzo pants softly moulded the contours of her still youthful figure, seemed similarly cool and relaxed as the heat of the day gave way to the humid warmth of the evening.

A succession of excellently prepared Provençal dishes based on locally-caught seafood and colourful regional vegetables and fruits provided a superb meal, that was accompanied by a delicious rosé wine. Darkness fell with Mediterranean swiftness and the constant chirping of the crickets in the garden provided background music to the murmur of conversation at the table.

"You have never visited a perfumery, mademoiselle?" Michel's father found it hard to believe that any human being could lack such a singular experience. "We must change that at once. I shall arrange for the car to bring you to our maison in Grasse tomorrow. My son will have the honour of showing you the premises and the scents we create."

Holly thanked her host warmly, noting that Michel's enthusiastic response was counterbalanced by the thin line of his mother's lips pursed in disapproval. She was more than happy to accept the invitation, not only to see the perfumery itself but also because she knew that Michel had to be there too; she did not relish the thought of spending the day at La Mouette alone with the baroness.

Towards midnight, dinner was over, coffee and cognac drunk, cigars and cigarettes smoked, and the guests rose to take their leave. On her arrival the previous evening Holly had found that she had been placed in a wing of the house as far from the family's own quarters as possible. With hindsight the tactic was obvious. Nevertheless politeness decreed that she should play their game while under their roof and she bade Michel a friendly good-night. With his chaste kiss on her lips she went to her room.

Bright light was streaming through the open shutters when she awoke the next morning. Although it was late, she lay for some minutes contemplating the pleasures of the day to come and, despite a guilty conscience, enjoying the fact that she did not have to get up to see to Rose. It was the first time they had been parted overnight and she missed her little daughter greatly, but she shuddered at the thought of bringing her to La Mouette!

After showering, she rang through to the kitchen as she had been instructed to do and a maid appeared with coffee and freshly-baked brioches. The Galliards clearly did not believe in communal breakfasting. At least she had been given a room with a balcony, albeit facing the gardens and the mountains, so she took the tray outside and enjoyed her breakfast in the sunshine.

She had just finished when the phone rang to inform her that a car had arrived to take her to Grasse. She slipped on a short-sleeved beige linen jacket which matched her sleeveless dress. Not wanting to look like a tourist she chose an elegant pair of black high-heeled sandals. A matching clutch bag completed her outfit, and feeling both cool and confident she descended the steps in front of the villa to where a chauffeur-driven Mercedes was waiting.

Although it was only mid-morning, the surface of the road was already shimmering in the heat. Thankful that the car was air-conditioned, Holly leant back in the soft upholstery and relaxed. The driver took the Route Nationale before turning off for the long climb upwards into the Alpes-Maritimes to reach the little town of Grasse. On either side of the road rippling fields of purple lavender stretched as far as she could see. At the touch of a button Holly lowered the window and a sweet, heady fragrance filled her senses. She breathed deeply, taking in the magnificent scent which had made this little town world-famous.

On their arrival at the perfumery the chauffeur ignored the visitors' car park, already crammed with coaches and cars from all over Europe, and drew up at a side entrance instead. He jumped out to open the car door for Holly, but before he could do so Michel strode from the building to greet her. Casual yet businesslike in a pale grey suit with an open-necked white shirt, he must have been watching from his office for her to arrive.

"Bienvenue à notre maison!" He kissed her cheeks in

welcome. "Let me get you something to drink. It's so hot. Would you like some water? Or iced tea? Orange juice perhaps?"

He was nervous, she could see, and she laughed as she shook her head, declining all his offers. She had already noticed with amusement that it would be an inexcusable faux pas to refer to the perfumery as a factory; it was a maison, a house like a fashion house, and, as with haute couture, the products it created were one of the world's greatest and most ancient luxuries.

She listened with interest as Michel personally conducted her around. On every stage of the tour they were accompanied by friendly but respectful employees. The company was, as he explained, like a big family with posts sometimes being passed on from generation to generation.

They began by inspecting the big vats where tons of blossoms were mixed with wax to extract their essential essences. Holly could see huge piles of flowers – roses, jasmine, lily-of-the-valley and mimosa – and he told her how the petals were mixed with imported fragrances of oriental origin such as musk, patchouli, cedar wood and sandalwood.

"Do you use synthetic ingredients as well?" She had read that many perfumes were chemically produced.

"No, we incorporate only natural essences," Michel replied. "That is our philosophy which makes the House of Galliard so exclusive and our fragrances so beautiful." He opened a door for her to pass into the next room. "This is our distillery. The fragrances being distilled here are for some of the great couture houses – Dior, Nina Ricci . . ."

"They are made here?" Holly was surprised. "I thought they made their own perfumes."

Michel smiled. "We help them create the scent they want. Then, if they wish, we make it and supply it to them in metal containers. All they have to do is bottle it in their own well-known flacons, name it, package it – and of course quadruple the price," he added wryly. "But naturally we are proud to make our own perfumes too. Here –" he reached for a glass bottle from a wooden rack which reminded Holly of the chemistry laboratory at school. He dabbed a drop of the colourless liquid on the inside of her wrist with the stopper. "This is one of our latest creations. What do you think?"

"Mmm, lovely," Holly murmured as a warm but fresh and elegant fragrance filled her senses. "It's light and young, but it has a very distinctive air about it. I'd recognize it anywhere. What is it called? Did you compose it?"

"Mon Dieu, no," Michel smiled. "It takes years of training plus inborn talent to become a nose, a 'nez' as we call them. The noses are our most valuable employees. They can detect one scent in hundreds. We totally depend on them to create our products. Not the sort of thing I learnt at business school! I deal with the marketing side of the company." He lifted her wrist to his nose and inhaled. "I love this fragrance too, but unfortunately it did not meet the requirements of our customer – you remember, the firm that had the presentation where we met? They chose the scent we both disliked."

Holly smiled. "I'm glad they did, otherwise we might never have started our first conversation."

Michel looked intently into her eyes. "I'll order this perfume to be bottled specially for you. It hasn't got a name, it isn't on the market, and I'd like you to wear a fragrance that no other woman has got." He bent his head over her wrist and breathed in the scent again, then, oblivious of the fact that they were not alone, gently kissed the spot.

Leaving the distillery they passed through the packaging and sales departments where noisy crowds of tourists were buying perfume at reduced prices. Finally they reached the manager's office where François Galliard awaited them. Charming and dapper as on the previous evening, he insisted on inviting them both to lunch at one of his favourite eating places, an open-air restaurant in the busy centre of Grasse. It was mid-afternoon before Holly found herself seated in the Mercedes again for the return journey to La Mouette.

On reaching the villa she went straight to her room and lay on the bed in darkness, the shutters closed against the pounding heat outside. The day had begun hot and the temperature had continued to climb steadily. The tour of the perfumery followed by the excellent food and wine that Michel's father had ordered all combined to produce a drowsiness which she did not normally feel at this hour. She tried to marshal her thoughts.

She was seeing Michel in another world, his world. His family owned a company whose name was known throughout France. They had a luxurious property in an exclusive location, even the prices on the menu in the restaurant had made her feel dizzy, yet she knew he loved her and he seemed to want to share that world with her.

Thinking was hard. Her head was beginning to ache. She raised a hand and laid it across her brow. As she did so, a faint scent met her nostrils. It was the perfume he had dabbed on her wrist and its fragrance stayed with her as she slept.

She woke up with a jolt. A glance at her watch showed that it was nearly six o'clock. Was it day or night? Where was she? Why was she dressed? Someone was knocking. She raised herself on one elbow and stared round the room. Seconds passed before she remembered where she was.

"Un moment, s'il vous plaît. J'arrive."

She struggled to her feet and went to open the door, trying to straighten her dishevelled clothes and smooth her hair on the way. When she opened it, Michel was standing there, looking as fresh and bright as when she had first seen him that morning.

"I'm so sorry." She tried to suppress a yawn. "I must have fallen asleep when I got back this afternoon."

"You look even lovelier when you have just got out of bed. I'm sorry I woke you. I've brought you a present."

"How nice! Thank you." She unwrapped the tissue paper. It was a bottle of perfume. "Is it . . . ?"

"Yes, it's the scent you liked today. I had it made up specially for you."

The slim, elegant bottle of the palest blue glass had a plain white label. 'Pour mon amour', she read. 'For my love'.

"Oh Michel, no one has ever given me a present as beautiful as this before."

He took her in his arms and kissed her tenderly. "I'm sorry I had to work today, but I've kept the rest of the week free for us to spend together. We can do whatever we like. Well, perhaps not everything!" He eyed the bed with grin.

Holly laughed. "If we can't do that, let's go out for the day tomorrow like we do in Paris. It's heavenly here. I'd love to see more. And tonight? Let's eat out! Just the two of us."

His face fell. "I'm so sorry, darling, but that won't be possible. I should have mentioned it earlier. It's le quinze août, August the fifteenth. My parents have arranged a special celebration. In any case, we'd never get a restaurant table now. Everything has been booked up for weeks. We'll go out tomorrow night, I promise."

Holly sighed. She had forgotten the date. She knew that the Catholic Feast of the Assumption of the Virgin Mary was not just an important religious festival but a highlight of the social calendar. As every year, there would be family parties and fireworks throughout France. That meant she would have to face another formal dinner with Michel's parents and their friends.

Michel looked at her sympathetically. "We can try to get away, just for a while." His voice showed that he shared her disappointment. "I've got to go now and get out of this suit. I'll meet you for aperitifs." With another kiss he was gone.

By eight-thirty over twenty people had gathered on the terrace, drinks in hand, and a babble of French, English and Italian greeted Holly when she joined them. Michel was at her side at once and introduced her to some of the other guests, most of whom seemed to be neighbours occupying villas on the Côte for the summer.

Holly's glance took in the women's ornate gowns. Despite their familiarity with one another, they were dressed with such formality that she was glad she had abandoned her first choice for the evening, a light chiffon dress, in favour of an evening trouser suit in emerald green. The jacket was cut narrowly in the style of a man's dinner jacket to reveal the curves of her body. Its shimmering satin against her sun-tanned skin, and the severity of the cut relieved only by her gold ear-rings and sandals, made heads turn in her direction, the men's in admiration, the women's in envy.

Holly could sense Madame Galliard's eyes following her every move and was not surprised when she found her place card in the dining room set between those of two elderly Frenchmen who ignored her completely and conversed over her head. Michel was seated at the far end of the table next to the only other young woman present, the daughter of an Italian shipping magnate, an attractive brunette in a gorgeous pink Cerruti gown, so stunning in its simplicity that Holly thought it must be the work of Cerruti's young designer Giorgio Armani. She was relieved when, three hours and six courses later, the dinner drew to a close. After coffee and liqueurs Madame Galliard rose to her feet and, as at a signal, the assembled company followed her like a flock of chattering birds onto the terrace.

Darkness had fallen and Holly was surprised to see a large number of cruise ships, motorboats, yachts and other sailing craft gathered out at sea with chains of lights strung over their masts and festooned with coloured lanterns.

"What are they all doing?" she asked Michel.

He smiled. "Just wait. You'll see."

No sooner had he spoken than the fireworks began. Patriotic cockades of red, white and blue exploded into the sky over the water. Then a new tableau, cascades of gold and silver against the black backdrop of the night, brought cries of wonder from all sides. Even before it had faded away, huge chrysanthemums burst into luminous radiance, blues turning into greens, reds into oranges and purples into pinks. Michel had moved close behind her. His arms encircled her, his hands covered her own on the parapet and she felt the warmth of his breath on the nape of her neck.

"Mmm, lovely," he breathed into her ear. "You're wearing my perfume." His voice was husky when he spoke again. "I want you wearing only my perfume."

Holly did not trust herself to reply. Those around them gasped as yet another fountain of rockets hit the sky to fall like multicoloured stars reflecting vividly on their upturned faces.

"Let's get away from here," he whispered, and without waiting for an answer, grasped her hand and pulled her away from the balustrade where their places were immediately filled. Behind the backs of the other guests, he took her down a flight of steps and into the gardens. "Round here." He led her away from the house and towards the swimming pool. "They can't see us here." Holly pulled off her sandals that were clattering on the tiles. She felt the terracotta beneath her bare feet, smooth but still warm from the heat of the day. Michel tossed his jacket onto the ground and knelt on it, drawing Holly down towards him. She could see only the outline of his form against the night sky, hear only the explosions of the fireworks and the ensuing cries of the spectators.

Very slowly he leant forward and kissed her lips. He raised one hand to release the clasp that held her dark hair so that it fell like a curtain around her shoulders, then drew his finger in a line down her neck to her cleavage. He watched spellbound while she undid the buttons of her jacket one by one and shrugged the green satin from her bare shoulders. She unfastened the clasp of her delicate lace bra and when it fell away he reached out to touch her breasts. Pulling off his shirt he lay down and drew her close to him.

"I want you to wear only my perfume," he whispered again.

Holly slipped off her satin trousers, casting aside the wisp of her panties. They explored each other, each seeking to give the other pleasure in secret places and finding delight in doing so. Time and place were forgotten in the spell woven between them. When his cool firm body covered her own, her hands felt the muscles of his back ripple as they moved rhythmically together and her crescendo of excitement matched his own until they finally became one.

"Holly, je t'adore," he breathed in her ear as they lay peacefully at last. Her eyes rested on the midnight sky, now lit by thousands of tiny stars. He began caressing her again, but she gently broke away and sat up. The fireworks display must have finished long ago. She could hear the buzz of voices on the terrace. "Michel, we must go back. We'll be missed. Your parents . . . "

"Pouf! Mes parents!" She recognized Arlette's French gesture of nonchalance. She could see that he was not in the least concerned about his parents, but he rose reluctantly and helped her to her feet. They dressed as quickly as they could in the darkness. Since people were taking their leave when they re-entered the house, their absence seemed to have gone unnoticed. Holly did, however, register a pointed glance which Madame Galliard threw in their direction as they mingled with the departing guests, shaking hands, kissing cheeks and exchanging au revoirs. She wanted to escape as soon as possible. She longed to be alone, away from the clamour of voices, to go through the happenings of the day in her mind, to try to sort out her feelings.

In her bedroom at last she went onto her balcony. She could dimly make out the gardens below her window, and beyond them the pool where Michel had made love to her, glinting like glass in the moonlight. She would always carry the memory like a precious jewel in her heart, one which she could bring out, look at and turn over in her hand whatever the future might bring.

What would the future bring? His world, in which he felt so at home, was not hers. She had hated the dinner party and found the thought of further similar events unbearable, yet he had been completely at ease. She could face the enmity of his parents, but could he? She knew that Michel's father would also turn against her if she became more than just a charming visitor. They had other plans for their only son and heir – marriage to a girl of wealth and breeding, not one struggling to support a child.

Was he prepared to anger and disappoint his parents for her sake? Or was she just another of those delicious luxuries to which he was accustomed? She remembered the girl in the Cerruti dress who had been hanging onto his every word. Michel could have any woman he wanted. Did he really mean it when he said he loved her? Could she trust him?

Holly put her head in her hands. She had hoped for so much from this holiday but nothing was going the way she had expected. She had been so happy in his arms, yet now she was unsure. Perhaps she was over-tired. Perhaps she was missing Rose. Perhaps everything would be different in the morning when they would spend the day together. Perhaps . . .

She turned and went into her room, closing the shutters behind her, and only a trace of her perfume lingered in the night air . . .

TWENTY-FOUR

North Yorkshire, Spring 1964

. . . The letter is brief.

The London College of Fashion is pleased to offer you a place on the three-year Diploma course in Fashion Design, beginning on October 5th, 1964.

Details follow about fees and accommodation but Holly reads no further. One sentence is enough, one sentence that is the fulfilment of the dreams she has cherished for as long as she can remember.

She can hardly believe that her application has been successful although her tutor was adamant that she should submit her work. At the interview in London she was ill with nervousness, cowed by the other applicants radiating self-assurance with their home-counties accents and their stylish clothes. Her responses were so timid that the examiner had to ask her to speak up, robbing her of the little confidence she had and any hope of ever being accepted.

And now, unexpectedly – this! She unfolds the letter to read the magic words again, then places it on the table for Nick to see when he arrives. He has gone to visit his mother and sister at the Hall before coming to her flat. It would have been nice to go with him but the place will be full of relatives – masses of aunts and uncles come to celebrate his mother's birthday, he has told her, a family affair, so maybe it is better for her not to intrude. At his twenty-fifth birthday party in July he wants to introduce her 'officially' to his family. 'Officially'. She has not asked but she can guess what it means.

She hears his car outside and by the time she has checked her hair and makeup he is in the room, sweeping her into her arms, swinging her round, covering her face with kisses.

"I've made it, Nick! I've made it! I've got a place at the London College of Fashion!"

The plans she has been making all week to tell him over a romantic dinner, the table set with candles, the steak and the red wine she has saved up to buy, all are forgotten.

"That's fabulous! Oh Holly, my dear, sweet, wonderful Holly! How fantastic!"

He takes her in his arms again and kisses her lips, long and tenderly. She looks into his laughing grey eyes. He is the first person she has told and in sharing her news with him she has doubled her joy.

"Come and sit down for a while. I'll just put the steaks in the pan. You must be hungry. Would you like a glass of wine?" she calls gaily from the kitchen.

"Love one." His long loose form is sprawled on the sofa. "And I'm starving. You've no idea how ghastly Mother's birthday 'do' was. Nothing decent to eat, all my old aunts there wanting to know when I'll be qualified, and Georgina with some stuffy solicitor she's going out with. I hope to God she doesn't marry him."

"I'd like to meet Georgina again."

"She'll be at my party in July."

July! She can hardly wait. "By then I'll have finished my pre-dip course and be getting ready to go to London," she says proudly, coming into the room with two glasses of wine.

"To Holly Barton! Britain's top fashion designer!" He raises his glass.

"To us!" She is sipping her drink when a smell of burning wafts in from the kitchen. "The steaks!" She races to save them. When they have eaten, they sit holding hands.

"I can't believe you're coming to London in October. For three whole years."

"Nor can I. It hasn't sunk in yet. I've got so much to do first – apply for a grant and a place in a hall of residence – I could never afford a flat – and then . . ."

"Just a minute," he interrupts her, "you're going to live

with me, aren't you? I mean, that's the whole point of your coming to London. So we can be together."

His voice is raised. She notices that the wine bottle is empty though she has drunk less than two glasses herself. She tries to speak calmly.

"Nick, I'll see you every day if I can, but I've wanted to study in London since long before we met. That's the reason I'm going there."

"Oh, so I'm not important any more!" He sounds like a petulant child.

"Of course you are. I'm sorry, I didn't put that very well. It's just that the money I got from the sale of the house after Mum died is nearly used up. I'm taking a job on the post to see me through the summer holidays, but after that I'll have to live on my grant. I don't think my course will leave me time to earn much on the side so I've got to keep my costs low."

"But I have enough for both of us. You can live rent-free if you move in with me."

"You know I couldn't accept that. And it's not really your money, is it?"

"What do you mean? Of course it's my money!"

"Yes, but where does it come from? Who pays the rent?"

"Well, there's my grant, but that's only a pittance. The rest comes from home."

"By 'home' I suppose you mean your mother? Nick, I can't live off your family, surely you can see that. I have to support myself. That's what I've been doing ever since Mum died."

She can see that he is irritated. "Let's not quarrel. We can talk about it tomorrow."

He gets to his feet, then sways before steadying himself with one hand on the table. She realizes that he must have been drinking at the Hall before he arrived. "Sorry." He gives her a boyish grin. "That uncle of mine, making me drink that damned brandy. Let's go to bed now."

"Nick," she begins tentatively when she is lying in his arms, "you will be careful won't you? It's not a good time of the month for us to be making love. Perhaps it would be better if we didn't . . ."

"Of course I'll be careful, darling." He is stroking her cheek, looking into her eyes. "I always am, aren't I? Trust me. You know how much I love you. I'd never do anything you didn't want. I couldn't." And then his lips meet hers.

Somehow she knows, even the morning after, that this time things have gone wrong. Six weeks later she goes to see a doctor in a nice part of Middlesbrough with leafy avenues and big bow-fronted houses near the art college. The elderly GP reminds her of Flo's father. He is kindly but the news is bad.

"Let him get his own way, did you, my dear? Well there's not a lot we can do about it now. But you're a healthy girl, so the baby should be fine. Now don't you go trying any funny business! It's against the law for a start and you could do terrible damage to both yourself and the child. Best let nature take its course. Stand by you, will he?"

Holly mumbles an incoherent answer and leaves the surgery in tears. She knew the truth beforehand, but there was always a tiny backdoor of hope left open. Now that has closed and the reality of the situation is more than she can bear.

When she gets back to her flat she makes some tea and tries to think clearly. The letter of acceptance from the college is hanging from her pin-board, mocking her. In a burst of anger she rips it off, tears it up and throws it into the bin. There is no hope of doing the course in London now. She has got nothing, no one except Nick. She longs to see him. He will know what to do. They shared her joy; now they will share this, too. He has never stayed away for seven long weeks before, but he is coming on Saturday, the first time since that fateful weekend. She will tell him then.

His face is crimson. "What? Are you sure?"

They are standing in her little sitting room. He has not even sat down but she could not hold back the news any longer. She nods. He curses and lets himself fall onto the sofa, his head in his hands. She wants him to take her in his arms but he does not look at her.

"How could I be such a damned idiot?"

She sits down beside him. "Nick, it's not just your fault. It's mine as well. I should have stopped you. We're both in this together. We've got to see it through. After all, it's our child . . ."

He puts one arm around her shoulders but his head is still bent. She cannot see his face. "I've got to think," he mutters.

"What is there to think about? It's happened and there it is. It's just come a bit early that's all. I won't be able to go to college in London now but we'd surely have wanted to have a child one day . . ."

"Will you stop calling it a child!" His voice is brutal, ripping through her.

She is stunned. This can't be Nick, her sweet, loving, impulsive, generous Nick. She stares at him, unable to speak.

"I'm sorry, Holly. Just give me a minute." His head is in his hands again.

She finds her voice at last. "It's alright. I was in a terrible state myself at first. I'll make us some coffee."

"Haven't you got anything stronger?"

"Sorry, no."

When she comes back with two mugs of coffee he is standing by the fireplace and for the first time since she told him the news he smiles weakly at her, a flicker of that boyish grin she loves so much.

"Thanks. Just give me a while."

He sips his coffee. She forces herself to stay silent, to give him the time he needs to assimilate the new situation. It has taken her nearly all week, a week in which she has cried so much that there are no tears left inside her now. She waits. She must stay calm, be practical, not let her emotions carry her away. This is the first time their love has been tested. If they come through this together it will strengthen the feelings they have for each other.

"You're sure it happened then?"

"Absolutely. There's no other possibility, is there? After all, I don't see you that often." This time it is she who gives him a rueful smile.

He does not respond. "So – seven weeks. That's not too bad. In that case . . ."

"What do you mean, 'not too bad'?"

He takes her in his arms at last. The grey eyes look deep into hers. He is holding her tightly, as if to cushion her against a blow. "My darling, you don't honestly think you can have this baby, do you?"

She stares into his face. "Of course I can. What else . . . ?"

"Holly, my sweet. Don't be so naïve. I'm sorry, but neither of us is in a position to bring up a child. You've got your college place, it's what you've always wanted, and I have to take my finals yet. It's going to be years before I'm earning enough to start a family."

"I'm not being naïve at all. Oh Nick, don't you see? This is our child. Of course I'll give up my college place to have the baby! I'm young. I can study later. I can work until you're qualified and then, when you're earning you can support me. It won't be easy but we'll manage. Others do."

He pulls away from her roughly. "Maybe they do, but do you think that's the sort of life I want to live? Stuck in a tiny flat like this for years and years with a baby, nappies drying in front of the fire, no money to spend? We're both too young for that!"

She cannot see him for tears. "You don't want me to have the baby?"

His arms are holding her again. "I don't want you to ruin your life."

"So what do you want me to do? Get rid of it? It's against the law."

He makes her sit down on the sofa, then sits beside her, taking her cold hands in his. She sees the scene in the farmhouse kitchen again, when he told her about her mother's illness. He is talking about death again.

"Listen to me, please, Holly. A friend of mine at university had the same trouble." She winces at the word. "His girlfriend was pregnant and he was at his wits' end about what to do. He got the address of this doctor in Islington. His girlfriend went there and that was that. All very hygienic, properly done, no back-street messing about. She was fine afterwards, honestly. Of course it wasn't cheap but –"

"– and that's what you want me to do?"

"It won't be as bad as you think, Holly. I can take you back to London tomorrow, we'll find out the address, get you an appointment and I'll look after you till it's all over. I'm nearly a doctor, you know." He is smiling, reassuring her, willing her to agree. "Then you can go to college in October and nobody will ever know."

"But I'll know. And you'll know."

"Yes, but one day when you've got your diploma and settled down in the job you want, then you can have a child and you'll forget all this. I know this is all a bit much for you now, but believe me, my darling, it's the only way."

"I don't . . . know . . ."

"Look, I'll leave you to think it over for an hour or two. I have to drive over to the Hall and help Mother with some tax forms she doesn't understand. I'll be back by six. Will you be alright on your own?" He kisses her cheek.

She nods miserably. She has never felt so alone.

When he has gone, she gets up wearily and takes the coffee mugs into the kitchen. She opens the bin and finds the bits of the torn-up letter from the London College of Fashion. They are damp and crumpled but she smoothes them out and arranges them so she can read the words again.

She wonders whether she will be able to put the pieces of her life together again as easily.

TWENTY-FIVE

Côte d'Azur, August 1969

During the remaining days they spent at La Mouette Michel seldom left Holly's side. The time seemed too precious to lie by the pool or on the beach at Cannes. Often they set off to explore the surrounding countryside, driving up tortuous Alpine roads past orchards of peach trees, vineyards and olive groves. In villages perched on mountain tops they ate outdoors in little restaurants where the midday sun shining through the vine leaves overhead dappled their clasped hands on the tablecloth. They talked, ate, drank, walked and swam together, but he did not make love to her again.

Their last day came. They had been to see the Picassos in St Paul de Vence and had begun the long drive down serpentine roads towards the coast. A brief summer shower had passed as suddenly as it had begun and Michel lowered the hood of the Alfa Romeo. After the oppressive noonday heat, the cool freshness emanating from the pine trees that lined their route was delicious. Holly breathed deeply, detecting scents of wild thyme and rosemary mingling with the fumes of the car in front, a mixture quite peculiar to the Côte d'Azur, she reflected. No other region combined the glories of nature with the pleasures of civilisation so perfectly. Since Roman times its people had known how to celebrate the art of living.

Michel's thoughts were more mundane. "We're running out of petrol," he announced, bringing her back to the twentieth century with a jolt. "Let's stop and fill up in Monte Carlo. Then we can have a look round Monaco."

Holly was thrilled. She would have felt that something was lacking if she had returned to Paris without visiting the principality. Michel seemed to sense her excitement because he stepped on the accelerator and the car sprang forward, zigzagging through the bends.

Monte Carlo was everything she had expected and more. The towering apartment blocks of the rich and famous crammed together in the tiny bay, vying for sea views, had turned the former pirates' hideaway and smugglers' haunt into a mini Manhattan. She could hardly believe that only a few kilometres lay between the elegant shops which would have graced Fifth Avenue or Bond Street and the medieval villages through which they had just passed.

They parked near the casino, a huge, elaborate building on cliffs overlooking the sea. When they went inside, Holly caught her breath at the sight of the ornate anterooms. Although it was still afternoon, the lights of the vast chandeliers reflected on gold stucco, polished marble and rich mahogany, an ambience of wealth and luxury more consistent with the nineteenth than the twentieth century.

Michel showed her round, lowering his voice as if they were inside a church. In a way, Holly thought, it was a church, a temple to the god of money. She eyed the people entering the saloons with curiosity. "Surely they can't be gambling at this time of day?"

Michel smiled at her remark. "Why not? But of course the really serious business goes on in the evenings. I once watched an American oil baron lose a fortune at roulette and still give a ten-thousand-franc tip to the croupier."

She felt uneasy in this place. "Let's go outside."

When they emerged into the bright sunshine she was delighted by the beauty of the gardens with their palm trees and exotic blooms. They walked on past luxury hotels till they reached the harbour, crowded with private cruisers and motor launches so large that they made the few sailing craft in their midst look like model yachts.

"How strange. It's the middle of the holiday season but lots of the boats look empty. I would have thought they'd be out at sea – you know, being used," Holly added awkwardly, aware that once again she sounded like a stranger to this world.

Michel put his arm round her as they leaned over the harbour wall, looking down. "Chérie, if you can afford a mooring here, you don't have to take your holidays in August when everybody else does. And even lying here, the boats are still being used."

"How come?" She looked puzzled.

"Most of them are for representation, for business interests, at least that's how their owners declare them for tax purposes. They are being written off as they lie here and probably making lots of money that way." She looked shocked. "Ma petite Holly," his hand stroked her hair, "you still have a lot to learn about the world."

She did not reply.

They rounded a corner and almost by accident found themselves standing in front of the palace. It was everything a royal castle should be. Perched on a promontory with battlements, towers and turrets, its flags flying, it looked like a toy fort. There were toy soldiers too, Holly noticed, as the uniformed guardsmen outside marched to and fro with great panache and ceremony.

They joined a crowd of tourists being held at a respectful distance by several gendarmes. To judge by their excited shouts and gestures, something was about to happen. At that moment a black limousine swept past them and vanished through the gates, its windows darkened so that they were unable to make out its occupants. The onlookers, who had been hoping to catch a glimpse of Princess Grace, started to disperse with mutters of disappointment. Michel seized her hand and said impulsively, "I want to buy you a present!"

"What? Here? You don't have to do that. This is about the most expensive place on earth."

"You're worth it."

He led her down a narrow street lined with boutiques. The names they passed were synonymous with luxury: Dior, Gucci, Hermès, Bulgari, Balenciaga. Holly managed to steer him past the jeweller's shops and in consequence they found themselves looking into the windows of the great couturiers. The clothes did not bear any price-tags but she knew that, even though they were from the prêt-à-porter collections rather than haute couture, they were far beyond anything that she could afford. She gazed in the window of one of the boutiques. The boat-necked, sleeveless dress in bright pink satin on display had a short fussy jacket with gold buttons and three-quarter-length sleeves. It was the epitome of what she herself would neither have designed nor worn.

Michel appeared behind her. "What are you looking at that for? It's awful. Come and look at this instead!"

He led her further along the street. The boutique bore the name Chanel. In the window there was a single black dress, cut on the bias to just above the knee with no ornament other than a white camellia at the waist. "That looks good. I could really see you in that."

Holly stood transfixed. "Good? It's brilliant," she said softly. "Coco Chanel is my idol. I really worship her. You know, she was designing in the thirties, then she went to Switzerland during the war and didn't design for fifteen years. But then Jacques Fath, one of the famous designers in Paris in the fifties, said that women were only fit to wear clothes, not design them. Coco Chanel was so furious that she came back and reopened her business and she's been designing successfully ever since. I think that's because only a woman can know what other women really want."

"Maybe you're right. The only way to find out is to go in and see."

Before Holly could stop him, Michel had entered the elegant black and white boutique and was asking whether she might try on the dress that was in the window. While it was being taken off the display dummy, she protested weakly.

"Michel, you can't possibly . . . I really couldn't . . ." But he just smiled and took no notice. She entered the spacious fitting-room and took off her denim shift. Even as she slipped the black dress over her head she knew it was going to be perfect. She looked at herself in the mirror and fell in love with it. When she emerged, Michel's eyes shone with admiration. Even the vendeuse, pin cushion in hand, found nothing that she could possibly alter and exchanged meaningful glances with Michel. She knew who would be paying for the purchase.

Then, just as Michel was flipping open his chequebook, something snapped in Holly's brain. She felt like a parachutist in freefall who suddenly pulls the ripcord. She looked at the price tag: she and Rose could live on that sum for two months. She knew it would make Michel happy to buy the dress for her, but what would be *her* price? She heard her own voice, as if another person were speaking. "No, I'm afraid it's not what I really want, thank you."

The vendeuse stared at her in amazement; she evidently thought she was either stupid or mad. Holly did not trust herself to look at Michel's face. She went back into the fitting-room, quickly took off the dress and put on her own clothes.

They left the shop in silence. She knew he was hurt. As they walked back to the car they passed through the casino gardens. A couple was coming towards them. The man was wearing a dinner jacket and the woman a red cocktail dress, but it was her magnificent necklace of diamonds which caught Holly's eye. She had no doubt the jewels were genuine, yet the wearer seemed quite unconcerned about parading a fortune in the street. Holly realized that she had seen no poor people in Monaco, no scruffy rucksack tourists, no families with noisy children, no beggars, no gypsies as in other parts of the Côte d'Azur. This was a place for the rich to be among the rich. She gripped Michel's hand so strongly that he looked down at her in surprise. "I'm sorry about the dress. It's something I can't explain right now. Can we go somewhere else?"

He stopped and bent to kiss her lips. "I think it's time we got out of here. I've planned to take you somewhere special tonight for our last evening." He smiled into her eyes. "And this time I won't take no for an answer."

When they reached the medieval village of Eze, perched in

a fairytale setting high on the cliffs, with quaint stone houses, winding alleys and breathtaking views, Holly thought she had never seen anywhere so beautiful. At the restaurant Michel had chosen they were led to a table set alone, overlooking the sea. The slight mistiness which so often marred the coast in summer had dissipated and the air was so clear that the blue of the sky met the azure of the water in a line drawn by an artist's pen. Fishing boats and yachts, cruise ships and tankers seemed to have been painted onto it. To the west, the evening sun was beginning to cast pink, orange and red rays across the heavens; the next day would be hot too but they would no longer be there.

When they had taken their seats, Michel leaned across the table and took Holly's hand in his. "I don't want this to end."

"It's been wonderful," she said softly. "Spending every day together. No work, no worries, just us."

His dark blue eyes looked into hers. "Let's spend every day together, always. Marry me, Holly. I love you. Will you marry me?"

She drew a deep breath. "Michel, I love you too. I love being with you, I love everything about you, but . . ."

"But?" He had withdrawn his hand and a puzzled frown creased his brow.

"I don't feel I can commit myself at the moment. I'm sorry. I know I'm hurting you by saying this, but I don't want to make any promises I can't keep."

"Is that why you wouldn't let me buy you the dress?"

Holly nodded. "Yes. If I'd let you do that, it would have meant . . ."

"It wouldn't have meant a thing!" he interrupted. "Do you think I'd have asked for something in return? Surely you don't think that?"

She shook her head. "No, of course not, but I would have been committing myself even more than I already have. I just don't feel ready for that yet."

"I know you haven't felt at home here on the Côte," he began slowly. "I noticed that, and especially today in Monaco.

- 251 -

And my mother hasn't been very welcoming either. I'm sorry." Holly could see that despite his hurt and disappointment he was trying to understand her feelings.

"That's not your fault."

"Yes it is, in a way. I brought you here, not just for a holiday but because I wanted you to see where I have my roots, so you could get to know me better. It doesn't seem to have worked out that way."

"Oh Michel, don't say that! I've had a fantastic time and I feel I know you far better now than when we were in Paris. Of course I wish your mother approved of me, but that isn't really the problem. It goes deeper than that."

"Is it connected with your work?"

"Partly. Somehow I just can't see where I'm going. The Montefiori contract runs out next year and they may want to take a different designer then. And I can't work for Arlette forever. In any case, it's hardly a proper job, I'm more like an overpaid assistant than anything else. I can't base my future on that, and I've got to support Rose. It's a responsibility that frightens me sometimes."

"But there's your own label." He pressed her hand again. "You're just starting to be successful! You're becoming known. Your designs are so great. And if you do what Maurice suggested and open a shop . . ."

"He made it all sound so easy, but it's not. Michel, I've always been absolutely hopeless at figures. Maurice wants me to draw up a business plan but I don't know how! And even if he lent me the money to get going, I've no idea of book-keeping, taxes and all that!"

"All that!" Despite her distress, he was forced to smile. "You're right. It is a lot and it isn't easy. But at least you realize that and aren't going into business with your eyes shut hoping it will all work out, like some people do. You can't do everything yourself. You are the creative head of the business, but you need someone else to handle the commercial side."

"Like who?" She could see where this was leading.

"Like me!"

"Michel, I can't let you."

"Why not?"

"Because you have your work for the perfumery."

"Pouf!" The familiar gesture once more. "I can easily draw up a business plan for you. And as for the books, I can do them at the weekend. It's hardly a global enterprise, is it?" He smiled again. "At least not yet."

"But Michel, I can't let you."

"We're back to where we started, aren't we? You mean you can't commit."

She didn't answer.

"Your work isn't the real problem at all, is it?"

She shook her head.

"Has it got anything to do with Rose's father?"

"No! I never want to see him again!"

He looked at her closely, studying her face. "It's got to do with England, hasn't it? Was there somebody there . . . ?" He broke off. Involuntarily she had caught her breath. His face darkened at once.

When he spoke again, his voice was shaking with anger. "I love you, Holly. I've asked you to share my life with me. If you can't accept that . . ."

He was on his feet. "We're leaving. There's no point."

She could see that he could barely keep his emotions under control. She rose and he led her back to the car.

During the drive back to La Mouette they did not exchange a word.

In Deauville the cool breeze off the Channel carried the promise of rain. Heavy clouds lay low on the horizon. Holly shivered and pulled her jacket tight round her body, wrapping her arms around herself to hold it there. Arlette joined her on the terrace of Beau Rivage, knotting a silk scarf at her neck. It fluttered in the wind as the two women made their way down through the gardens and onto the beach. The tide was receding rapidly leaving a wet expanse of sand strewn with shiny pebbles and shells. Their shoes left deep impressions that filled with water, a trail of little pools that followed them as they walked.

Holly had returned to Paris with Michel the day before. Their departure from La Mouette had been as she had expected. Michel's father had kissed her cheeks heartily and pressed her in the warmest of tones to visit them again; his wife had not seconded that invitation. With a formal hand-shake and a thin-lipped smile she had taken her leave of them in the evening and had not risen to see them go the following morning. Michel had barely spoken to her during the flight from Nice and had returned to his apartment in Paris. They had not arranged to meet again.

Holly sighed and looked out to sea, a swelling grey mass of water, so different from the Côte. She recalled the sparkling azure of the water, the deep green of the mountains, the brilliant white of the villas, the glowing reds, oranges, pinks and purples of the flowers – geraniums, oleander, bougainvillaea, jacaranda. Its colours were painted indelibly in her memory. Its scents of wild thyme and rosemary, lavender and pinewood lingered in her nostrils.

Yet she was glad to be in Deauville again. Until she had seen the little figure running to greet her, until she had swept her up into her arms and hugged her dearly, she had not realized how much she had missed Rose. The sea air had done her good and she had grown. Her skin was golden and her green eyes shone with vitality. Holly had held her close, wondering whether she could ever bear to be separated from her again.

After the excitement of their reunion, Rose was taking her afternoon nap. When she woke up, they would leave for Paris and their holiday would be over. Holly tried to suppress the thought of all the work that would be waiting for her on her return. She turned to her friend at her side.

"How can I thank you and Maurice for looking after Rose? I can see she's had a wonderful time. She looks fantastic."

"We've enjoyed having her so much. She's welcome to come and stay whenever she likes." They walked on in silence until Arlette spoke again. "Holly, something happened while you were away. It was in the papers and I feel you should know." Her voice was serious. Holly looked at her in alarm. "It's Julien. He's been arrested for possession of drugs."

Holly's heart lurched at the mention of his name. This was the first time either of them had spoken it for over two years.

"It seems he was caught buying a large quantity of cocaine. His flat was searched and the police found quite an arsenal of other drugs as well, far more than one person would use. They are still investigating the case, but he may end up being charged with drug-dealing."

"What's going to happen to him?"

"If they can prove the charges, he'll go to prison. Otherwise he'll have to pay a very heavy fine. Either way, he'll never be able to work in banking again."

"Less than he deserves," Holly retorted bitterly. "It's you I'm sorry for, Arlette, for the disgrace he's brought on your family."

"I stopped regarding Julien as part of my family two years ago," her friend replied. "Now what about you? I'm dying to hear all about your trip to Provence."

When Holly had finished, Arlette stopped and looked at her keenly. "Ma chère, you've told me all about your holiday, all the places you went to and all the things you saw. But, "she paused awkwardly, "you haven't said very much about Michel. Why hasn't he come with you today? Is something wrong?"

"He said he had a lot of work to catch up on for tomorrow."

Arlette was not deceived. "What has happened between the two of you? I know he loves you. It was obvious on your visit here, even Maurice noticed. We both think you're made for each other. You haven't split up, have you?"

Holly slipped her hand through Arlette's arm and they continued their walk. "He asked me to marry him."

Arlette stopped again, her eyes wide with astonishment. "But that's wonderful news!" Suddenly her brow furrowed. "You didn't refuse him, did you?"

"I couldn't accept."

"But why not? When he was here, I could see you were in love with him. What's happened between you?"

Holly could not meet her gaze. She stared out to sea instead. "I love everything about him. He's fun to be with, and exciting, but at the same time so gentle and kind. I love just being with him. We like all the same things. We can talk for hours and never get bored. He's fantastic with Rose too . . . " Her voice trailed off.

"But?"

"If I marry him, I'll be committing myself and I just don't feel I can."

"Did you tell him this?"

Holly nodded miserably. "Yes, he took it very badly. He's hardly spoken a word to me since."

"But there is more than that, isn't there? Did you tell him everything?"

Holly shook her head. Suddenly she felt ashamed. Until now she had not even told Arlette the whole truth.

"A long time ago I loved someone and he loved me. He was everything I'd ever dreamed of," she whispered. "So sweet and loving and kind. I thought he was perfect and I trusted him and then he hurt me so much. And then something terrible happened, the worst thing that's ever happened to me in all my whole life." She was crying now. "I couldn't go through that again, ever. It would kill me."

Arlette turned to face her. The beach was deserted now, the tide far out. "When Maurice asked me to marry him, I felt like that. I loved him, but the past was holding me back. I was clinging to my memories of all I'd lost. But Henri was dead and my darling Virginie too. That life was gone forever. That's why it was time for me to go forward and make a new life with Maurice." She paused and thought for a moment. "Holly, in a few weeks' time, when you've completed the Montefiori designs, why not leave Rose with me and take some time off to sort out how you feel."

"You mean go back to Yorkshire?"

"If you think that will help you, yes."

"I haven't been back for over four years." A gust of wind arose, carrying her next words away, over the sand and across the sea. "Maybe it's time to go."

TWENTY-SIX

North Yorkshire, October 1969

Flo hugged her friend affectionately, "It's so great to see you again. I could hardly believe it when you said you were coming, even if it is only for a few days. I thought nothing could tear you away from Rose and your work in Paris – but here you are!"

"Well, Rose is staying with Arlette and Maurice in Deauville for a week. They love having her and the sea air does her good, so I thought I'd grab the chance to come over here and see you and the moors again."

A slight look of puzzlement flickered in the blue eyes that were watching her across the table. Holly could see that her deliberately casual remark had raised questions in her friend's mind, questions such as why she had suddenly returned to Yorkshire after four years, why she had come without her child, and why she had chosen to arrive in the middle of the autumn term when Flo's work as a teacher meant they would not be able to spend the days together. Flo must have guessed there was a deeper reason for her visit but she had not asked, knowing that Holly would tell her when the time was right.

"Have some hotpot." Flo lifted the lid off the big iron casserole and a delicious smell pervaded the room. "My mother was convinced we would starve if she left us here without any food so she made this before she left. She doesn't trust my cooking and I'm afraid to say she's right."

Holly passed her plate. It was strange to be staying at the Westburys' home again. Outwardly little had changed. The comfortable house with its unpretentious furniture was exactly as she remembered it, just as outwardly she herself had changed little. Inwardly, though, she was a far different person from the lonely unhappy girl who had sat at this table over six years ago. She had not realized how different until now.

"It's absolutely delicious. You must tell her. It's a pity I won't be seeing your mum and dad." Dr Westbury and his wife had left the day before her arrival for their annual autumn walking holiday in the Lake District. Holly recalled how kind Flo's parents had been to her after her mother's death, but in a sense, she was relieved that she and Flo would be alone together. She did not feel like making conversation about her present life in France when the past was uppermost in her mind.

Flo was having similar thoughts. "Actually I'm rather glad they've gone. Not just because Dad really needs a break – he works so hard – but it's not easy living at home again when you're used to having your own place. Mum and I tend to cross swords now and then." She sighed as she got up to put the pot back on the stove. "When I left York, I had to give up the flat I was sharing with two other girls there. Mike and I are doing up the farmhouse now his father has moved out. Nothing has been done to it for years, since his mum died in fact, and it's a time warp in there, pure fifties. We want to get it perfect so we can move in after the wedding. Now that I'm teaching near Ainsley it seemed like an unnecessary expense to rent a flat for only a few months, so here I am, back at home." She grinned. "But that's not the only reason I'm counting the days till Christmas."

"Tell me about your work at school." Holly could feel herself starting to relax. The good food and the warmth of the open fire were making her drowsy. It had been a long day, in which she had flown from Paris-Orly to London and taken the train from Kings Cross to Darlington where Flo had picked her up in her car.

Flo's face lit up. If Holly had ever had any doubts about her friend's choice of profession, they would have flown now. "It's only a little village school, but that's what I like about it. The children come mainly from the farms, some of them really high up on the moors." For a brief moment Holly saw herself as a child again, dragging her bike out of the stables in the cold air of a dark winter's morning to ride to school. "They are really sweet, not like some of the town kids I had to deal with in York. I teach the youngest class, the five-year-olds. They've got so much life in them, they're so curious about everything, so interested. I hope they stay that way," she added wistfully.

"With you as their teacher, I'm sure they will."

"It's hard work sometimes just getting them to listen," Flo laughed, "especially on Monday mornings. They all want to talk at once." She rose to her feet, starting to clear away their empty plates. "Look Holly, I'm ever so sorry but I've still got some material to prepare for the craft lesson tomorrow, otherwise it'll be a complete shambles. Is it alright if I leave you on your own for an hour or so?"

"Of course. You do whatever you want. I'll deal with the washing up and then I think I'll go outside for a while and walk off your mum's hotpot. A breath of fresh air would do me good after all the travelling I've done today. I won't be long."

"Then take the torch that's hanging near the back door with you. It's pitch dark out there now, even though it's only October. See you later. Don't get lost!" she joked as she disappeared upstairs to her room.

When Holly found herself in the square she saw that Flo had been right. A thick blanket of unbroken cloud hung low overhead, blocking out whatever light the moon and stars might have given. The street lamps oozed a yellowish glow that was sucked into the surrounding gloom. The air was damp and cold. She shivered and turned up the collar of her coat. Her footsteps rang out eerily on the cobbles as she walked down the High Street. The shops were just as she remembered them: first the butcher's, then the greengrocer's, after that the co-op and then the café. All were closed and silent. No one passed her. Only a solitary car with dipped headlights edged its way around the Market Cross that stood like a lonely sentinel where the main roads met, the one snaking up onto the moors and to the sea, the other stretching inland, to York and beyond. It was hard to imagine that in a few hours the little town would come to life again with children chattering on their way to school, housewives bustling in the shops, lorries and buses, delivery vans and cars jostling for parking spaces and jamming the narrow streets.

She made her way uphill to St Nicholas' church. Even in the darkness she could see the great stone tower silhouetted against the sky. Then, as she rounded a corner, she saw light glowing behind the tall gothic windows and was drawn towards it. She pushed open one of the heavy doors and peeped inside. A group of people, men and women, young and old, were standing in a semi-circle at the far end of the nave. Suddenly the organ began to play. A man in their centre raised a baton and their voices broke into song. It was evening choir practice. She slipped noiselessly inside and sat in a pew at the back, in the shadows. They must be rehearsing for Harvest Festival. The hymn was one which she knew and loved. Happy memories from her childhood flooded back as the chorale of voices rose in a crescendo that hit the huge vaulted roof then died away, leaving the last notes echoing round the empty church. The choirmaster seemed to be satisfied and the group broke up. They were leaving now, talking and calling goodbyes. She went out before them, knowing where her steps would lead her.

A wind sweeping down from the moors was starting to disperse the clouds. In the moonlight Holly could make out the skeleton shapes of the trees in the Applegarth, and the dark line of the hills beyond. She switched on Flo's torch and picked her way through the tombstones till she came to the one she was looking for, the one that marked the spot where Elizabeth Barton lay. She bent down and read the simple inscription it bore. She felt in her coat pocket for a handkerchief and tried to wipe away the streaks of grime and tufts of moss that had settled there, but without success. Perhaps it was better to leave it so, at peace, and not disturb the traces of the passage of time. She rose, switched off the torch and remaining standing at the grave in the darkness.

Had she really known the woman who lay beneath this stone? They had lived together for so many years, but had they truly shared each other's hopes and fears? The Elizabeth who had loved and lost Philippe would forever be an enigma to her. She wished they had been closer, and yet, whenever she had had a problem, her mother had always been there to listen. In her quiet way she had never said much but had managed to help her find the solution for herself. Suddenly she had the feeling that she was not alone and knew for certain that, this time too, she would make the right decision. A sense of calm spread through her. She switched on the torch again and quickly made her way back to the doctor's house.

Flo was in the kitchen as she entered. "Gosh, you look frozen. Come on in. I've got the stuff ready for the kids in the morning. Now, what about a nightcap? What do you fancy? Wine or cocoa?"

Holly grinned. "I drink wine so often at home that a cup of cocoa actually sounds quite exotic."

"When I make it, it probably is. I can even manage to burn water." Flo poured milk into a pan and put it carefully on the stove. "Just like old times," she said later as she smiled at Holly over the rim of her mug. They were curled up at opposite ends of the big sofa in front of the fire. "Remember all the things we used to tell each other? All the secrets?"

Was it a chance remark or an invitation? Perhaps both, Holly thought. She sipped the hot chocolate before she replied. "It's good to be here, good to see you again, but there's another reason why I've come." Flo's eyes never left her face as she told her friend about Michel's proposal.

"How much does Michel mean to you?" Flo asked softly.

"I love him, but I loved Nick too and he loved me and you know what happened. I've tried to forget, but I can't. I'm too scared of getting hurt again."

"And why have you come back?"

Holly took a deep breath. "I have to see Nick again. I want to find out why he acted as he did, ask him how he could do that to me if he really loved me."

Flo put down her mug on the hearth and stared into the fire, concentrating. "Right," she said at last. "What we need is a plan of action. When's your flight back?"

"On Sunday. I have to be at work on Monday."

"Well, it's Thursday now. That gives you exactly two days. This is what you do. Take my car for the day tomorrow." She raised her hand to silence Holly's protest. "You'll need it to get around and it'll do me good to take the bike to school. I have to lose a few pounds if I'm going to get into that wedding dress you made me. At lunch time I'll ring Georgina at her school in York and find out what I can about Nick – how he is, where he is, what he's doing et cetera. There may be a chance you can see him on Saturday before you leave the country." She turned and faced Holly. "What do you think?"

Holly was speechless. Everything had become so simple. "That sounds fantastic. I don't know what to say."

"Rubbish." Flo got to her feet, stretched and yawned. "That was nothing. Just try having twenty little kids to organize."

"I don't envy you. One is enough for me."

Flo lifted up the telephone and placed it beside Holly on the sofa. "I have to go and get my beauty sleep now. Up here in the wilds of Yorkshire we don't keep the same hours as you Parisians. I'm off to bed, but before you come up give your friend Arlette a ring. Let her know you got here alright and tell her to give Rose a big hug tomorrow morning from her Auntie Flo."

Holly smiled. "You bet I will."

A loud bang woke Holly up the next morning. She looked around, unable to make any sense of her surroundings. The bedroom seemed strangely familiar. For a moment she thought she was reliving the night her mother died, but then slowly everything fell into place again.

She looked at her watch in the dim light. It was nearly eight o'clock. The noise she had heard must have been Flo slamming the front door on her way to school. She threw back the bedcovers and went barefoot downstairs to the kitchen. A note in her friend's handwriting was lying on the table beside a bunch of keys.

She yawned as she put the kettle on. She had not slept well. The wind had risen to gale force during the night, howling in the chimney, beating on the roof and rattling the glass in the window frames as if nature were mirroring her own disquiet, but now, outside at least, the storm had abated. Beyond the wet garden she could see a pale sky washed with aquarelle blue and torn wisps of cloud disappearing to the west. In the east thin fingers of sun were feeling their way over the hills.

A piercing shriek made her jump. The kettle was boiling. She made some tea and sipped it thoughtfully, trying to decide where her day would take her. The hot strong liquid seemed to flow straight into her brain, and by the time she went upstairs to wash and dress, a plan was forming in her mind.

The engine of Flo's battered mini spluttered into life when she turned on the ignition. She engaged gear and reversed gingerly onto the road, smiling to herself as she remembered Flo's note instructing her in the strictest terms to drive on the left. She drove carefully through the town and then, getting the feel of the car, accelerated to take the bends that led uphill towards Black Ridge Farm. She did not know what had made her decide to go there first, but she felt she should start by going back to the beginning.

The distance seemed further than she remembered. Had she and her mother really lived alone on this wild bare moorland for so many years? At last she drew up in the lane in front of the farm. When she switched off the engine, the silence was overwhelming. She got out and went to lean on the five-barred gate. The farmhouse lay before her, nestling into the hillside. A spiral of smoke climbed out of the chimney into the clear air and two of the upstairs windows had been flung wide open. The front door was painted green and, as she watched, a woman came out carrying a baby that she placed in a pram outside. There must be other children too for there were bicycles leaning against the stable wall. A multi-coloured array of washing strung on a line across the yard, stirred in the breeze. A swing hanging from the branch of a tree moved slightly in unison and behind it, in the paddock, two ponies were grazing in the sunlight. The house had an air of peace and contentment.

The woman was at the door again, watching her, clearly wondering who she was. For a moment Holly debated whether she should open the gate, cross the yard as she had done so many times before and introduce herself, but she dismissed the idea. She had no place in these people's lives, nor did she wish to see the inside of the house again. She wanted to remember it as it had been: the kitchen where her mother had sat sewing when she came home from school, the front room which they had used only at Christmas, and her bedroom where she and Flo had exchanged their secrets. She could not risk losing those memories. It was enough to know that Black Ridge Farm was a home, a place of warmth and happiness again. She got back into the car and the woman on the threshold watched as she drove down the lane again.

Without thinking she found herself taking the road to Ranleigh Hall. Georgina was living in York, recently married, Flo had said, and Lady Marianne had moved into a nursing home there over a year ago. The Hall had been placed on the market with planning permission for conversion into flats, a country house hotel or an old people's home. Holly slowed the car as she drove up the long winding drive. She was preparing herself for the worst. The days when one family had inhabited such a mansion, the days of servants and gardeners, shooting parties and balls, luxury and leisure, had gone forever. The war had brought that era to an end. The Ranleighs had tried to stem the tide, struggling on into the sixties, but in the end they too had been forced to abandon a doomed way of life.

She took the last turn and suddenly the Hall was towering before her. The sight of the great house had always made her catch her breath, but this time she sat motionless behind the wheel, too shocked to get out of the car. The windows on the ground floor were completely boarded up. The massive door had been smeared with paint, daubed with words she did not try to decipher. Huge holes gaped in the upstairs windows where vandals had hurled stones to break the panes. The carefully-tended lawns and flowerbeds had become a tumble of weeds, and grass was sprouting between the flagstones in the porch. A noticeboard advertising that the property was for sale lay on its side amongst the shards of glass, jagged bits of wood, dead leaves and broken flower pots that littered the front steps.

Holly did not know how long she sat there; she only knew that a deep sadness came over her. In many ways the Hall had not been a happy place. Lady Marianne had suffered there, losing both her husband and her health. Despite their family's wealth, Nick and Georgina had not had a loving, secure childhood. Yet the old house had not deserved this end. She hoped that an investor would be found. Any development would be better than the desolation which lay before her.

She felt physically sick. It was an effort to turn the car and drive back onto the main road. Her eye fell on the little clock in the dashboard and she was shocked to see that it was past twelve. She had not had anything to eat all morning, no wonder she was feeling giddy. She stopped at a roadside café where she ordered coffee and scrambled eggs. When she had eaten, she felt ready to face the next stop on her journey of reminiscences.

The road over the moors ran along a high ridge from which she could see far down into dales where grey stone villages and solitary farms dotted a patchwork of green, yellow and brown fields and copses. Sturdy moorland sheep knee-deep in the heather watched her impassively as she drove by, occasionally wandering into her path so that she was forced to stop and wait until they ambled away. When she reached the top of the moors, the distant sea came into view, glinting in the sun.

She slowly descended Lythe Bank. The memory of the day when she had come here with Nick was so vivid that she felt she could have reached out to touch him again. She passed the spot where they had been forced to abandon his car, and on an impulse pulled into a space at the bottom of the bank. Where had he taken her from here? The cottage had not been far away. She knew it would hurt but she wanted to retrace their steps, wanted to see if something of the magic of their first night together still lingered there.

She found a path leading off the road and into the trees. Whereas they had been dark and leafless then, their branches now were richly clad in scarlet and orange, russet and gold, yet the way seemed familiar. She could almost feel the cold seeping through the soles of her boots once more and the warmth of Nick's hand holding hers. She plunged further into the woods, but with every step her feet sank deeper into the mud. Brambles tore at her clothes and scratched her face until a dense tangle of undergrowth finally barred her way.

There was no sound of the stream. There was no sign of the cottage. Like a fairytale castle it had vanished into the forest. She was forced to give up. She made her way back to the car. Perhaps it was better that she should not find it again.

She parked the car on the sea front and leant over the rusty railings on the promenade. The tide was almost in. Seaweed and driftwood had been tossed high onto the beach, vestiges of last night's gale, and the sea was still rough. Huge grey breakers came rolling to crash into white foam at her feet. The air was filled with salty spray. When she closed her eyes, she could feel Nick's arms around her again, she could taste their first kiss.

The afternoon sun was dipping below dark clouds on the horizon. Another storm was threatening. She watched in fascination as, minute by minute, it drew closer. The breeze sharpened into a strong wind blowing in gusts from the north.

She remained there, bare-headed, gazing at the spectacle of sight and sound until raindrops, cold and hard as bullets of ice, sent her running to the shelter of the car. The day which had begun in sunshine was drawing to an early close. The headlamps cut through the driving rain as she drove in darkness over the moors. The bleak landscape had seldom seemed so forlorn. At last she reached the Westburys' house where a light in the hallway gave out a welcoming glow. Flo must be home now.

"Hi, come on in. How was your day? I've opened some wine. I thought you might need it." Flo managed to hug her, take her wet jacket, hang it up and press a glass into her hand all at the same time.

Holly sank down onto a kitchen chair. "I feel exhausted and you're the one who's been working, not me. How was your day?" she countered, afraid that an answer to Flo's question might release the turmoil of emotions within her.

Glancing at the pallor of Holly's face, Flo took her cue. "Incredible as ever. You'd never believe some of the things little kids can get up to," and she recounted a few anecdotes which had them both shaking with laughter. Putting two plates on the table she said, "Hotpot again, I fear. But never mind, like a good wine, it's supposed to get better the longer you keep it."

"Well?" Holly looked expectantly at her friend. They had taken their places at the table as on the previous evening and Flo was calmly proceeding to eat her dinner.

"Well what?" Only the blue eyes shining across the table revealed that she was teasing.

"Come on, Flo. I've got to know. Did you manage to speak to Georgina?"

Flo laid down her knife and fork. She was savouring the suspense of the moment. "Yes, I phoned her at her school in the lunch break." She took a sip of wine.

"What did she say? Did you ask her?"

Flo finally took pity on her friend. "Nick's in Newcastle. He passed his finals and is doing further training in plastic surgery at the Royal Victoria Infirmary there."

"Newcastle? But that's only about fifty miles from here! I thought he'd be in London or even abroad somewhere."

Flo felt in her pocket and pulled out a scrap of paper. "Here." She pushed it across the table.

"This isn't . . . ?"

Flo nodded. "It is. It's his phone number." She picked up her knife and fork again. "Georgina said you can ring him any time after nine tonight."

Holly looked at the row of figures, saying nothing.

"Are you going to tell him what happened?"

Holly thought for a moment. "Perhaps."

Flo did not press her to say more and after clearing the table went off to bed, leaving Holly alone with her thoughts. What would she ever do without dear Flo, she asked herself, the only one to have stood by her in her darkest hour . . .

TWENTY-SEVEN

North Yorkshire, Spring 1964

. . . Flo is sitting on the sofa in Holly's flat, her blue eyes filled with concern. "Are you really sure you're going to go through with this? When I read your letter, I just couldn't believe it. I had to come and see you."

"I'm so glad you're here." Holly sits down beside her friend and squeezes her hand. "You're the only person I've got to talk to. I haven't told anybody else." She pauses and wipes her swollen eyes with her wet handkerchief. "There's really nobody else to tell. Thanks for coming, especially now." She knows that Flo should be back at college now after her Easter vacation.

"I couldn't go to York and leave you on your own." Flo looks closely into Holly's face. "Are you sure you want to have the baby?" she asks again.

"Oh Flo, I couldn't bear to get rid of it. It's our child, Nick's and mine. I couldn't just kill it. We loved each other so much, we were going to get engaged in the summer." Tears well up and spill down her pale cheeks again.

"Did he actually propose to you?" Despite her pity for her friend, Flo asks the question, knowing it will hurt.

"Not exactly, but he said he'd introduce me officially to his family then and I took that to mean we'd be getting engaged. He told me he loved me. I trusted him. Oh Flo, how could it end like this?"

"Are you certain he won't support you?"

"When I told him I wasn't going back to London with him he got really mad and we had an awful row. He drove off in a furious hurry and I haven't seen him since."

"Does he know you're going to keep the baby?"

"No. I said I needed more time to make up my mind, but

I've thought it over again and again. I couldn't go through with an abortion." She bursts into tears again.

Flo puts her arm around her shaking shoulders. "Haven't you heard from him at all?"

"He sent this." Holly pulls out a thick envelope from behind one of her mother's candlesticks on the mantelpiece and hands it wordlessly to her friend.

"But there's money in it." Flo is looking at the bundle of notes in her lap in amazement. "He sent you this?" she asks incredulously.

"Yes. A hundred pounds."

"And no letter?"

"There was a letter as well, with the address of a doctor in Stockton."

"You mean, where you should go for an abortion?"

"He wrote that he could understand that I didn't want to travel to London to have it done and that this doctor could be trusted to do everything properly. That's what the money was for."

"Have you got the letter?"

"No, I burnt it."

"Was that all it said?"

"No, he wrote all the same arguments that he made when he was here. And he even finished by saying that he still loved me! Oh Flo, how could he write that and ask me to do such a terrible thing?"

"So you're not going to see him again?"

"Never! Not after this. Sending me money! How could he do something so sordid? It makes me feel cheap and dirty."

"But Holly, are you absolutely sure you're going to keep the baby? It will change your whole life. It'll mean all sorts of difficulties . . . and you won't be able to go to college in London."

Her voice is defiant. "So I can't go there this year – but that doesn't mean I won't get there one day. Anyway, this baby is more important to me than that. It's mine, all I've got left now."

Her arms are folded over her stomach, defending her unborn child.

Flo hugs her tightly. "You've got me, don't forget that. I'll help you all I can."

"I know you will. I don't know what I'd do without you. But now your vacation's over you'll have to go back to York. I'll be on my own then."

"But how are you going to manage? What are you going to live on?"

"I'm going to finish my pre-dip course at the art college here. I can afford that. Then I'll get a job on the post for the summer. That pays good money so I can save a bit, and after that I'll find something else – working in a shop or a café, I suppose. The rent for this place isn't much. I'll manage."

"And that?" With a nod Flo indicates the envelope with the money Nick has sent.

"I'm going to put it all in the bank to buy things for the baby."

"When's the baby due?"

"At the beginning of January, the doctor says."

"And after that? How are you going to cope then? It's going to be so hard for you, working and bringing up a child on your own. You haven't got training for a proper job and there'll be two of you to support. And it may be 1964 but people can still be pretty horrible towards unmarried mothers, you know."

Holly turns on her friend, hurt and dismayed. "I thought you were on my side!"

"Of course I am, love! I just want you to know what you're letting yourself in for, that's all."

"I'm sorry," she smiles through her tears. "I didn't mean to snap. You're right to tell me those things. Don't think I haven't been through all the pros and cons a thousand times. I've thought about nothing else for the last fortnight. Maybe I'm being naïve, maybe I'll regret it, but I've made my decision and that's that."

Flo goes into the kitchen and starts unpacking a carrier of food she has brought. "Well, in that case let's start by cooking you a good meal! You want building up. You're going to need all the strength you can get. Now let's see if I can manage not to burn this . . ."

No one told her it was going to be like this. Not at the antenatal class, not in any of the books she read. She tries to breathe slowly, in and out, in and out, but another pain sears through her, forcing her to grit her teeth and clench her fists in agony.

"You're doing very nicely, dear." The elderly midwife looks kind but exhausted. A piercing scream comes from a woman behind a curtained-off section of the ward. It goes on and on, then seems to reverberate round the sterile room long after the woman has ceased wailing. "Now don't you worry about her. She's just having a bit of a hard time, that's all, but it won't be long now."

"What about me? How long will it be before my baby's born?" She does not think she can cope with another contraction. The hands of the clock on the wall have been dragging themselves through the hours since the early morning. It is now nearly two in the afternoon.

"It'll be a fair while yet, dear. You just relax and see if you can think about something nice. Imagine how proud your husband's going to be when he sees you with your little one." The wrinkled hand pats the sheet over her distended abdomen and moves away.

She longs to scream. If she can let out all the pain of labour, maybe all the hurt inside her heart will go too. Nick should be here. He should be waiting outside with the other fathers-to-be, pacing the floor, praying that she and the child will survive this terrible ordeal. Instead she is alone. She was alone in the night when the contractions started. She was alone in the taxi coming here. She was admitted to the hospital alone, shaking her head when they asked her who the baby's father was. If she starts to scream now, she knows she will never stop.

Now another pain is coming, a huge wave of black water

towering over her, lifting her up, crashing over her head, roaring and pounding in her ears. She cannot breathe. She panics. She hears her voice shouting for the midwife, but nobody comes.

If only Flo were here. Flo, the only person she rang before she left.

Is it minutes or hours later? She is too weak to tell. All she knows is that a doctor is there, listening to the baby's heartbeat through her skin. The midwife is at his side. He is shaking his head. They converse briefly. She strains to listen and hears only the word 'operate'.

They are pushing her bed forward, banging it against the doorway in their haste, wheeling it into another room, calling in loud voices, throwing the covers aside. Someone in a mask is swabbing her stomach with a cold liquid. She is briefly ashamed of her nakedness before something hard is placed over her face and she is falling downwards into darkness.

When she opens her eyes, she is in a high white bed in a single room. Her mother was in a single room when she died. Is she going to die too? She feels nothing. Maybe death is like this. Someone is at her bedside – a young nurse who gently strokes her hand before she drifts into unconsciousness again.

Once more she awakes and this time the doctor is here. His presence reminds her of the pain she felt. Has he come to hurt her again? Why don't they just let her sleep?

They are waiting, she can tell. Waiting till she is ready. When she opens her eyes again, they bring her water to drink. They tell her that she has had an emergency caesarean section. The baby's heart stopped beating. They had to operate. She wishes they would stop telling her all this and bring her baby to her. Why are they taking so long? Why are they exchanging glances? Why is the doctor holding her hand?

"I'm sorry, my dear, there was nothing we could do. Your baby was a little girl but she was too weak to survive the birth."

She says nothing, just stares. This cannot be true. There

must be a mistake. They mean somebody else. Her baby was so strong, kicking and turning all these months, somersaults of joy for them both.

"Has the husband been told?" The doctor is speaking quietly over his shoulder to the nurse. She catches the words 'not married' in the reply.

She has to tell them that they are wrong about the baby. "But my doctor checked my baby's heartbeat regularly. He would have told me if there had been anything wrong. I'm sure . . ."

Her voice trails off. She is no longer sure of anything. The doctor is still holding her hand. "Perhaps it's better for you to know the whole truth, my dear. Your baby had a serious defect. Have you heard of spina bifida?"

She stares at him in horror.

"I'm afraid there was no way your baby could have lived. Perhaps one day we'll be able to save these children, but at the moment there's just nothing we can do. I'm sorry."

"Can I see her? Can I hold her in my arms just once?"

"It's better not. Believe me," he repeats, "it's better that way." She turns her head to the pillow to hide her tears. "We're going to give you something now to make you sleep." He squeezes her hand and leaves the room.

She does not want the injection but she has no strength to fight any more. Everything has been taken from her. She has been left with nothing and now, as the blackness closes in, they are even robbing her of her grief.

A nurse bustles in with a bright 'Good morning', takes her temperature and her pulse, gives her an injection and checks the dressing on her stomach. No words are exchanged. Then the young nurse of the night before brings her breakfast, soft bread and weak tea. Her eyes are sad and she whispers "I'm so sorry" when she puts the tray down, and then scuttles away as if she has broken some rule they taught her at nursing school.

Holly pushes the tray away. Why can they not just leave

her alone? Why did they not let her die with the baby? Her whole being, her body and her soul long for the child she has lost. She feels so empty. Her arms are empty, her body is empty, her heart is empty, only her soul is full of sorrow. Her mother, her home, the man she loved and now her child – all taken from her in one short year. How many useless, meaningless years lie ahead?

The door opens again. She turns her head away, but it is Flo. Then Flo is beside her, her arms around her, her head buried in Holly's shoulder, in tears.

"Oh Holly." She cannot go on.

Holly wants to comfort her but they weep together.

"So there was nothing they could do," she finishes, some time later when they are both calmer. "I've lost my little daughter." Her voice breaks. "I can't believe it. It's like a nightmare, but I can't wake up. They keep telling me that even if she'd lived, she'd have been severely handicapped. As if that somehow makes it all less terrible. The doctor said she had a 'defect' – as if she was a machine with a part gone wrong, not a person at all. How can they talk like that?"

"And you never saw her?"

"No, that's the worst bit of all. They told me it was better that way, and I was too weak to stop them. I wish I'd seen her. I wish I'd held her in my arms, just for a minute. I'd give everything to know what she looked like. I don't even have a photo of her, let alone a memory."

"I'm sure she was beautiful," Flo says softly. "Have you given her a name?"

"A name?" Holly looks at her friend through her tears. "No. I . . . I never thought . . . she never lived . . . she wasn't christened. I don't even know what they've done with her body."

"But she should have a name for you to remember her by."

"I'll never forget her. She'll always be my first child. I shall call her Florence Elizabeth."

"Oh Holly. That's a lovely name. Thank you for calling her after me."

"You're my dearest friend, Flo. I don't know what I would

do without you." Holly takes Flo's hand in hers.

"I wish I could do something for you. I feel so useless."

"Don't say that. You've helped me more than I can say. But I've got to face this on my own now. I wish I'd died with my baby, but somehow I've got to carry on."

"Maybe you can get a place at the London College of Fashion again. They'd take you next year, I'm sure."

They sit silently, hand in hand, each with her thoughts.

Then Holly slowly shakes her head. "I'm not going to apply there again. There's no way I can go back to any bit of the life I had. I couldn't face it after this."

"So what are you going to do?"

Holly's face is grim. There is a bitterness in her voice that Flo has never heard before. "All I want to do is get away from here."

TWENTY-EIGHT

North Yorkshire, October 1969

There was no mistaking his joy and excitement.

"Holly! I can't believe it! Is that really you? That's fantastic! After all this time! Where are you? How did you get my number?" His voice was exactly as she remembered it. The years seemed to fall away as she listened. When she told him that she was in Yorkshire, Nick at once suggested they should meet.

"Tomorrow's Saturday so I'll be off duty at the hospital for the afternoon. I have to go and see my mother in York but I could easily drive over to the Westburys' house on the way there. It'd be great to see you again."

Holly hesitated. Something advised her against seeing him again in Ainsley. It would be better to meet on neutral ground.

"There's no need for you to go so far out of your way. Isn't there some place near here that you'll be passing through? I could meet you there."

"Good idea," he replied cheerfully. "That way we'll have more time to talk. What about The George at Rothsby? It's just near the A1. I'll turn off there on my way down from the north and you can get to it via Thirsk."

The name of the town meant nothing to her, but she agreed at once.

"Fine, let's say three o'clock? Oh Holly, I just can't wait to see you again. Till tomorrow then."

He sounded smooth and confident. She had only time to say 'goodbye' before there was a click and the dialling tone returned. When she put down the receiver she found herself shaking.

It was barely half past two when she steered Flo's little car into the car park of The George Hotel. She had deliberately left the Westburys' house early. She wanted to compose herself before seeing him again. She wanted to be first at the venue.

When she looked at the hotel, a feeling of distaste swept over her. It was not the charming old English pub she had envisaged but a mock Tudor property run by a brewery chain. She wrinkled her nose at the smell of fried food and stale beer that greeted her on entering the restaurant, and chose a seat at a table which gave her a clear view of the car park. A youth who looked more like a student than a waiter wandered over and, ignoring the sticky menu propped behind the cruet, she ordered a pot of coffee.

She had dressed with care in a dark-brown trouser suit in fine cord from her latest collection, wearing it over a honey-coloured cashmere sweater that Arlette had given her for her birthday. She knew that the autumnal tones suited her; outwardly at least she looked serene and self-assured. Her eyes constantly scanned the car park. Her fingers shredded a paper napkin. This was ridiculous, she told herself. She could handle this. She had planned the meeting. She knew exactly what she was going to say. He was the one who should be nervous.

A black Ford saloon pulled up on the tarmac almost outside the window where she was sitting and Nick got out. She was taken completely unawares and realized she had been looking for the red MG he had driven so long ago. She watched as he made his way towards the door of the hotel. The easy grace of his movements and the casual elegance of his clothes had not changed.

He appeared on the threshold, running one hand through his curly fair hair tousled by the wind, and his glance fell on her. He was not nervous at all. The roles were reversed. His face broke into a broad smile and in a few long strides he was at her side. She rose shakily to greet him, then felt his hands on her upper arms, his lips on her cheek.

"Holly, at last! You're even more beautiful than I remembered!" His grey eyes looked down into her own.

Awkwardly they separated to take their seats on opposite

sides of the table. "I'm sorry about this place." He glanced round the room with a sniff of displeasure. "I should have thought of somewhere nicer but your call really took me by surprise. We can go to a different place if you like?"

"No." She shook her head. Their surroundings were unimportant. "It doesn't matter."

The waiter approached again and Nick ordered a coke. He waited impatiently until they were alone before he spoke.

"I honestly never thought I'd see you again. Not after we split up so suddenly. When you wrote me that letter saying you didn't want to see me again, there was nothing I could do except let you go. I was really cut up about it. I've missed you so much."

Holly could not speak. What was he saying? How could he talk about himself after all the pain he had caused her? All at once she began to fear that she might not be able to handle this after all. She had spent the night going over and over in her mind what she would tell him, but now that the time had come, the carefully-rehearsed phrases had flown out of her head.

The waiter brought Nick's drink and he half emptied the glass before he put it down and looked at her expectantly. He seemed about to speak. She knew she had to ask first, to stay in control, to keep the upper hand.

"Tell me what you've been doing. I hear you're a qualified doctor now."

"Dr Ranleigh at your service!" He half rose, smiling, and took a little bow. "I'm specializing in plastic surgery. That's why I'm up in Newcastle. Some of the best consultants in the country are at the Royal Victoria Infirmary." He felt in his jacket pocket and pulled out a rumpled pack of cigarettes. Holly was surprised. She did not recall that he smoked. "You don't, do you?" he asked, pointing the packet towards her. "Do you mind if I do?" She shook her head and he drew out a cigarette, lit it and inhaled deeply, flapping the air so that the smoke would not drift in her direction. "Sorry, bad habit, but it more or less goes with the job."

There were grey shadows under his eyes and lines on his face, but he went on to tell her about his work at the hospital with the same boyish enthusiasm she remembered from their first meeting on the moors so long ago.

"That means you're one step nearer to realizing your dream," she said when he had finished.

"My dream?" He looked at her questioningly.

"Yes, you once told me about it – helping people like the wounded in Vietnam. You said you wanted to use your medical skills to reduce some of the suffering in the world."

He smiled at the memory. "I suppose I did. Don't we all say things like that at that age? We're all idealists when we're young." He leaned forward, looking earnestly at her. "What about you? Tell me what you've been doing. What about *your* dream?"

She told him about her life in Paris, starting with her job as an au pair and how she had become Arlette's assistant, her designs for the Montefiori collections and finally her efforts to create her own label. He listened carefully, interrupting her now and again to find out more.

"Phew. That's fantastic. You've really done a lot to be proud of. This shop you want to open, where is it going to be? Are you going to stay in Paris? Are you there for good?" There seemed to be more behind his questions than just the desire to know her career plans.

"I haven't made up my mind yet."

"Maybe I can help you do that." His voice was soft and persuasive. His eyes sought hers.

"I've got to fly back to France tomorrow," she said quickly. "This is just a short visit. I wanted to see the moors and the coast again. Lots of things have changed since I left. I'm sorry about the Hall."

"What's there to be sorry about?"

"I went there yesterday. It looked so sad and abandoned."

"Well, it was never very much of a home for Georgina and me. Let's hope it fetches a decent price soon. Mother's splitting the money between the two of us to avoid death duties later on. It'll be just what I need to buy my way into a practice. My time at the RVI in Newcastle will be up next year and the London area is damned expensive."

"You're not coming back to Yorkshire?"

"Would you?"

"I suppose not," she was forced to admit. "I have to be where my customers are."

"Same with me. All my contacts are in London, and there's not as much demand for cosmetic surgery in the north."

"You mean facelifts and that sort of thing?"

He laughed. "Yes, I do. Don't look so shocked, I'll do my fair share of other work as well: kids with burns, people with scars and disfigurements, victims of accidents and so on. I'm not entirely without a social conscience, you know, but something has to pay the rent and London prices are astronomical." He stubbed out his cigarette. "And I have to think about settling down one day," he added meaningfully.

He reached out to take her hand but she withdrew it just in time. His voice dropped lower, taking on an urgent note. "I've never forgotten you, Holly, not in all this time. I tried to, God, I really did, but it was no good. I've had other relationships of course. Caroline and I were even engaged for a while, but I've never stopped thinking about you. Seeing you again makes me realize how much you still mean to me. We had such a great time together. It was fun. Let's see if we can make a new start. Put the past behind us and be like we were then."

She sat motionless, cold as ice. "I have a little daughter now," she remarked coolly. "Her name's Rose."

He looked surprised. "Are you married?"

"No."

A flicker of panic crossed his face. "How old is your daughter?"

"She'll be two in February." She could see him calculating, swiftly counting the months and years, then visibly relaxing.

"She's not ours then." It was a blunt statement rather than a question.

"She's not yours."

He did not notice the change of pronoun, that for her there was no 'ours' any more. This was what she had come for. This was the moment to tell him all the horrors that she had suffered alone. This was her chance to find out at last how he could have hurt her so terribly if he loved her so much.

She deliberately let it pass. There was no need any more.

He glanced at his watch. "I'm sorry, I've got to go. I can't keep my mother waiting any longer and I have to be back on the wards tonight. Let's see each other again soon, Holly. Georgina told me that your friend Flo's getting married at Christmas. We could meet again then and when I'm back in London, maybe you can fly over for the weekend. Let's give ourselves another chance."

He rose to his feet and at once the waiter was beside him with the bill. Nick handed over a ten-shilling note and told him to keep the change. When they stood alone again, he bent his head to kiss her lips but she turned her cheek to him instead.

"Goodbye, Nick."

"You have my phone number," he said softly. "I won't say goodbye, Holly. I'll say au revoir."

She watched from the window as he got into his car outside. It was starting to grow dark and he switched on the headlamps. They cut two bright arcs of light as he circled the car park, then they vanished and he was gone.

A low table was set for tea in front of the fire. The starched white damask cloth, the gleaming silver teapot and Mrs Westbury's best Wedgwood china welcomed Holly as she entered the sitting room. A dish of crumpets with a toasting fork lay on the hearth; their accompaniments – a pat of creamy butter and a pot of heather honey – were on the table, together with crumbly Wensleydale cheese, a rich fruit cake and slices of sticky parkin, the treacly dark gingerbread that Holly remembered from her childhood. "A real Yorkshire tea!" she exclaimed in delight.

"Comfort food." Flo came in from the kitchen carrying a

dainty jug of milk. "We're not counting calories tonight."

Holly sat down on the sofa, surveying the spread before her with relish. "Exactly what I need! How did you know?"

Flo speared a crumpet and held it in front of the flames. "I didn't. I thought I'd take pre-emptive measures. You never know where journeys into the past can lead you."

Holly poured the tea and sipped hers thoughtfully. Flo passed her a hot toasted crumpet and she spread it with butter and honey that melted and ran through the holes. It was delicious. The food was a special treat that demanded to be enjoyed for its own sake. They ate in a comfortable silence.

When she had gathered the last crumbs of cheese and fruit cake from her plate and drained her cup, Holly leaned back in satisfaction. Driving back after her meeting with Nick, she had tried to sort out her feelings, to make some sense of the turmoil inside her brain. Now her thoughts were clearing and she was deeply glad that Flo was there to share them with her. She knew her friend was waiting for her to speak first.

"He was there." She tried to keep her voice steady. "He looked just like I remembered him. The way he moved, the way he talked and smiled, nothing had changed." She paused. Flo was looking at her levelly. "He said he'd never been able to forget me. Oh Flo," the words came out in a rush now, "he even wanted us to get together again."

Flo's eyes never left hers. "It's what you want that counts."

"I wanted to hate him like I've hated him all these years. But nothing happened inside me. The hate somehow just wasn't there any more. Even when I saw him again for the first time, getting out of his car, he just looked so . . . " she searched for words, ". . . so ordinary. And when we talked, I realised there was never anything special about him at all. I never saw him that way before. I used to think he was perfect, but when I think back now, when I remember how he treated me, I think he was really just out to please himself most of the time. I was a fool to believe him when he said he loved me!"

"Maybe he did love you – in his way."

"Maybe he did. Maybe he still does. But it's not my way of loving. When he spoke of our relationship today, he said it'd been 'fun' and that we'd had 'a great time'. For him it was fun, but for me it was the most important thing in the whole world! How could I have been so blind?"

"Don't be too hard on yourself, love. Try to remember what it was like for you then. There you were – just eighteen - and then this really good-looking guy comes along, upper-class background, big house, flashy car, London flat, student doctor and so on – and actually falls for you! Any girl would have been head over heels in love with him, especially if she'd just left school, had never had a boyfriend in her life and never been further than the sleepy Yorkshire dale she grew up in! Then you lost your mum and your home and he was all you'd got! Don't you see, Holly? Nick was your knight in shining armour! He was your Lancelot coming to rescue you! When he came to meet you today, you probably thought he'd turn up on a white horse!"

Holly could not help smiling. "Not exactly a white horse, but I did expect to see him in his red sports car. It was quite a shock when he got out of a plain black saloon!"

"That's exactly what I mean. You wanted someone to admire and look up to, someone to take care of you. But he's an ordinary person, not a Greek god that you have to put on a pedestal. And don't forget, you're a Valmont. Your ancestors were nobility at the French court when the Ranleighs were still digging up potatoes – or whatever it was they dug up in the sixteenth century!"

"Turnips, I suppose."

They both had to laugh, but a moment later Holly was serious again. "I was going to ask him how he could leave me when I was expecting his baby and send me money instead. I was going to tell him about Florence and how she died. I wanted to know how he could do that to me." She was looking into the fire, speaking almost to herself. "But then I realized he didn't see any wrong in what he'd done. He was so relieved that Rose wasn't his, perhaps he'd even have been glad that the baby died."

"So you didn't tell him?" Flo asked gently.

"I didn't want to share my memories of Florence with him. She's mine. She'll always be in my heart. Without Florence I'd never have kept Rose. They're sisters in a way, they belong together."

Flo could only nod, too moved to speak.

"I made the same mistake with Julien. I was so lonely in France at first. I thought he knew best and that if I let him take charge, he'd take care of me. But I was wrong. When I wanted to assert myself, he wouldn't let me. And I paid the price."

"The world is full of Juliens, Holly, and they're on the lookout for women who aren't strong enough – emotionally, I mean – to look after themselves. But you've changed," Flo went on. "You're not the lonely insecure girl you used to be. You've made your way in Paris. Look what you've achieved. You've got every reason to be self-confident and proud of yourself. You don't need a man to look up to any more. You deserve an equal partner. Someone who loves and respects you and whom you can love and respect in return."

"I see that now. Coming back again has made me see that times have changed. Black Ridge Farm has changed, Ranleigh Hall has changed, your life is going to change as well, Flo. Life itself is change. So it's time for me to go forward and move on too."

"Yes, but when we move on, we take our memories with us. They make us into what we are. That's what makes childhood so important."

"My childhood wasn't perfect." Holly's face softened as she spoke. "Life was hard. Dad died so young and I often think that Mum and I never really knew each other, partly because she had to work so much to keep us both. But she was a product of her generation as well and I was only a child. If she were alive today, I'm sure we'd talk to each other quite differently from the way we did then. But in spite of everything, I always knew they both loved me and I loved them too. Nick doesn't care that the Hall is up for sale because it doesn't hold any happy memories for him.

In a way, my family was richer than his ever was."

Flo nodded. "Mine too, and you know, I think part of the magic has been the whole sixties thing. The sixties have been a good time to be young. New ideas, new music, new fashions, new freedom in the way people think and behave. Don't you think we were lucky to be growing up then?"

"Yes, but they're nearly over now. Only a few more weeks to go. I wonder what the seventies will bring."

The firelight flickered on Flo's face and Holly could see the happiness shining in her eyes. "Mike and I will be married and have a home of our own. We're going to be very busy, him working on the farm and me teaching at school, but we want to start a family in a year or two. How about you?"

"I've found a man who loves and respects me," Holly said quietly. And I love him too. Not the way I loved Nick, but in a way that makes me trust him and want to share my life with him."

"Michel?"

She nodded. "It won't be easy. His family doesn't accept me."

"Is that so important? You're not marrying his family!"

"True," Holly smiled. "And he loves Rose, so we'll have a family of our own." She drew a deep breath before she spoke again. "And I'm going to open a shop."

"A shop?"

"Yes, in Paris. One that sells exclusively *Holly de Valmont* designs!"

"That's fantastic! This calls for a celebration, don't you agree? I put a bottle of Dad's bubbly in the fridge, just in case, but I thought we should have the right music to go with it as well." Flo went over to the radiogram in the corner of the room and picked up a record that was lying on its lid. "So I bought this LP today. It's new out. 'Hits of the Sixties'." She slid the black vinyl disc out of its shiny cover. "The first track is a real oldie." She laid the record on the turntable, pressed a switch and the arm of the record player slowly descended to place the needle in the groove.

"It's by The Beatles. *Love me do.* Wasn't it one of your favourites?"

Lennon and McCartney's voices filled the warm room. Holly listened. The words held only sweet memories for her now.

Flo was handing her a glass of champagne, smiling.

"Here's to us."

Holly rose to her feet. She smiled back at her friend.

"To us – and to the future."

"Goodbye, sixties!"

"Hello, seventies!"

"Glad you came back?"

"Very glad."

Epilogue

Christmas Eve, 1969

The bells of St Nicholas' rang out joyously in the cold winter's air, their peals echoing throughout the dale. Inside the ancient church the guests had taken their seats, their hushed whispers and expectant murmurs mingling with the quiet playing of the organ. Beyond the stained-glass of the windows snowflakes were falling softly, while within, candles flickered in iron sconces on the stone walls, casting trembling shadows on pillars that rose to disappear into the blackness of the vaulted roof. Boughs of fir and pine filled the air with a warm woody scent, and on the altar, huge bunches of holly gleamed green and glossy in the candlelight.

The music stopped. The last chimes of the bells overhead died away. For seconds there was silence, broken only by the fizzle of a gutted candle. No one moved or spoke. Suddenly, the great organ burst into sound. To the magnificent strains of the Wedding March the congregation rose as one to its feet.

Holly could see Mike in the front pew, standing tense and nervous beside Dave, his best man. She watched him finger his unaccustomed tie and twitch the white cuffs that protruded from the sleeves of his new suit. Then he turned to look down the aisle and his face seemed to melt with pride, love and happiness at the sight of his bride.

There was a rustle of silk as Flo swept past slowly on her father's arm. For a moment her eyes met Holly's and sparkled with gratitude. Her lips parted in a radiant smile; she knew she was beautiful. The dress was perfect. She carried a bouquet of red roses with mistletoe and her fair hair peeped out from under a juliet cap like a golden halo.

Dr Westbury bent to kiss his daughter's cheek before

leaving her with Mike at the altar and joining his wife in the pew in front of Holly. Mrs Westbury, resplendent in dusky pink, raised a lace handkerchief to her eyes to wipe away a tear, and Holly saw her husband place a comforting hand on her arm.

The age-old marriage ceremony began and the congregation was asked to sit. As she took her seat again, Holly smoothed the fine ivory wool of her coat over her matching dress. Leah had made both to her own designs and she had worn them only once, ten days before, at a simple ceremony in Paris. This time too, she wore a pillbox hat of dove-grey suede over her long dark hair, and her gloves lay on the pew beside her.

The congregation had fallen silent. Flo and Mike were exchanging their vows.

"I, Florence Judith, take thee, Michael Alfred, to my wedded husband, to have and to hold from this day forward, for better or worse, for richer or poorer, in sickness and in health, to love and to cherish, till death us do part."

Mike's voice rang out strong and clear. "With this ring I thee wed, with my body I thee worship, and with all my worldly goods I thee endow."

As the lovely words of the timeless litany unfolded, Michel took Holly's left hand in his. Slowly he raised it to his lips and gently kissed the plain gold band that encircled her finger.

Printed by: Copytech (UK) Limited trading as Printondemand-worldwide,
9 Culley Court, Bakewell Road, Orton Southgate, Peterborough, PE2 6XD